# DISRUPT
## YOUR LIFE

Create your own kind of extraordinary through
the choices you make every day

By
Neryl East and Michael McKeogh

Text © 2019 by Neryl East and Michael McKeogh

All rights reserved. No part of this book may be reproduced or transmitted in any form or by any means, electronic or mechanical, including photocopying, recording, or by any information storage and retrieval system, without written permission of the authors.

ISBN: 978-0994329233

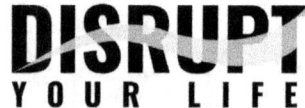

www.disruptyourlife.com.au

# Disclaimer

This book is designed to provide information and practical tips for readers. Advice in this book has been derived from the authors' experience and that of the individuals interviewed as part of this publication.

No warranties or guarantees are expressed or implied by the content in this book. You are responsible for your own choices, actions and results.

© Neryl East and Michael McKeogh, all rights reserved

# Acknowledgments

We would like to thank each person who has contributed to our lives and to the publication of this book.

To Briana, Connor and Abby, it can't have been easy to have a Dad so seriously injured and unable to always be the strong support you needed in your teenage years. You have become adventurous, free-spirited and courageous adults. Thank you for the support you gave me and for the joy you bring to the world. This story has shaped your lives too, and in your unique way, you have each pursued your own life disruption.

To the experts who contributed their insights to this book; Dr Jenny Brockis, Allan Parker and Sarah Boyd, thank you for your time and generosity in helping to create a bigger picture of what it means to bounce back.

To our families, we love and appreciate you and cherish the fact that your own stories are intertwined with ours.

To our friends—bike riders, paddlers and many others—we're so grateful for your support and involvement in our lives.

And for everyone who reads this book, we hope our story inspires you to think differently about the daily choices and actions that shape your life experience.

# Contents

Introduction ............................................................................................. 1
1. The lure of two wheels ................................................................... 3
2. Adventures on dirt ....................................................................... 15
3. Coming to a sudden stop ............................................................ 27
4. Memories that are best forgotten ............................................. 39
5. Homecoming ................................................................................ 51
6. The long road ............................................................................... 63
7. The next three seconds—insights from Allan Parker .......... 75
8. New friends and giggly goals .................................................... 81
9. Superpowers and a state of thriving—insights from
    Dr Jenny Brockis ......................................................................... 95
10. Anything is possible ................................................................ 105
11. The keys to bouncing back—insights from Sarah
    Boyd ............................................................................................ 117
12. Disrupting your own life ........................................................ 127
About the authors ............................................................................ 147

# Introduction

There are many stories about people who have triumphed in very challenging, even life-threatening, situations; circumstances that could be considered a life disruption.

Every case is different and yet there are recognisable patterns in how certain individuals respond.

Some have been diagnosed with fatal diseases and defied medical professionals by emerging in a fully healthy state.

Others have felt the impact of poverty or extreme disadvantage yet have gone on to become world leaders or icons in the business community.

There are those who have experienced unimaginable physical or emotional trauma and have thrived in their chosen career or life path.

Not everyone has results like these. You don't have to look far to see evidence that many people are crushed by the circumstances they encounter.

Appalling suicide rates, news reports of alcohol-related violence, divorce statistics… the list goes on.

On a personal level, you probably see negative comments in your social media feeds every day that indicate people's state of mind about their own problems or issues affecting their world.

What's the difference between those who rise above major challenges and those who let problems of any size derail their life? Is it one factor? Or a series of behaviours learned over time? Or are some people just lucky?

This is a story about one life disruption and what we learned from it.

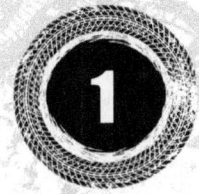

# The lure of two wheels

**Mike**
*Skinned elbows and witches' hats*

Is there something in your life you're passionate about—maybe a hobby or sport you started doing as a child and have carried through your life?

For me, unquestionably, that thing was riding motorbikes. I have to say *was*, because that's a key part of this story. But here's how it started.

My first memory of sitting on a bike was as an eight-year old at what was then called the Police Citizens Boys' Club, which morphed into the Police Citizens *Youth* Club when political correctness became a thing.

We lived right near the club at Engadine, a suburb on the southern edge of Sydney.

The big drawcard was that the club had what they called a driver-trainer section, where kids could hire small motorbikes and have a go at riding.

Was I any good to start with? I think "pathetic" would be the most appropriate adjective. I don't believe there was a worse rider than me in the group. And, as well as being hopeless on the bike, I had no mechanical abilities.

I could barely make the bike go forwards without jumping or stalling the engine. I fell off all the time; I'd break or bend various levers and dented the tank. There were constant repairs.

But that didn't matter. I loved it.

I was nine when we got our first family bike. Mum and Dad bought one little mini-bike that was shared between my brother, my sister and me.

That certainly was the start of something!

I'd like to say I had a meteoric rise to becoming a skilled rider, but even with the ability to now practise at home as well as at the club, my progress was slow. Still, I made up for it with enthusiasm.

The great thing about being in the club was that police officers would come to our sessions and give us training. They explained the road rules, showed us how to use stop and give-way signs and how to approach intersections.

They also trained us in what we called gymkhana riding—in a similar vein to what riders do on horseback—which involved tight manoeuvring around witches' hats on a dirt course.

That helped us learn to steer the bike quickly from left to right, to stop and turn, accelerate and use the brakes properly.

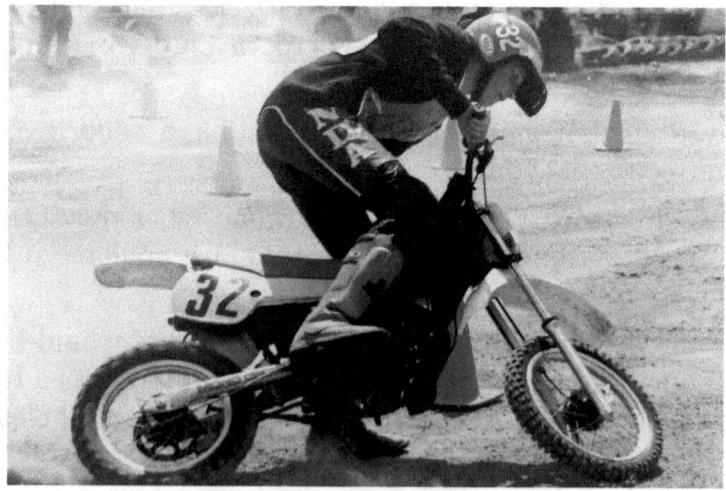

*Navigating the witches' hats. I was rider 32 in the club and that number stayed with me over the years.*

*1 | The lure of two wheels*

From there, we collectively progressed to managing a whole range of obstacles; climbing steep hills, riding over rocks and logs and taking our bikes through gullies. As you can imagine, this took time, patience and plenty of spills.

The club divided riders into A, B, C and D grades. If you were at the bottom of the heap as a D-grader, you had to ride in a specific area under strict control. The C-graders were allowed to go out with a group onto the nearby bush trails—still under close supervision. As you moved through the grades from B to A, you got to go on the faster trails that required greater skills.

No-one wanted to stay in D grade for long; we all wanted to do the really cool stuff.

As we progressed, we also learned tricks including jumps and wheel stands. These were great fun for a bunch of kids and also resulted in quite a bit of damage. It wasn't unusual for us to flip our bikes, always at a good speed, so we'd often go home with skinned elbows and bodies along with damaged bikes.

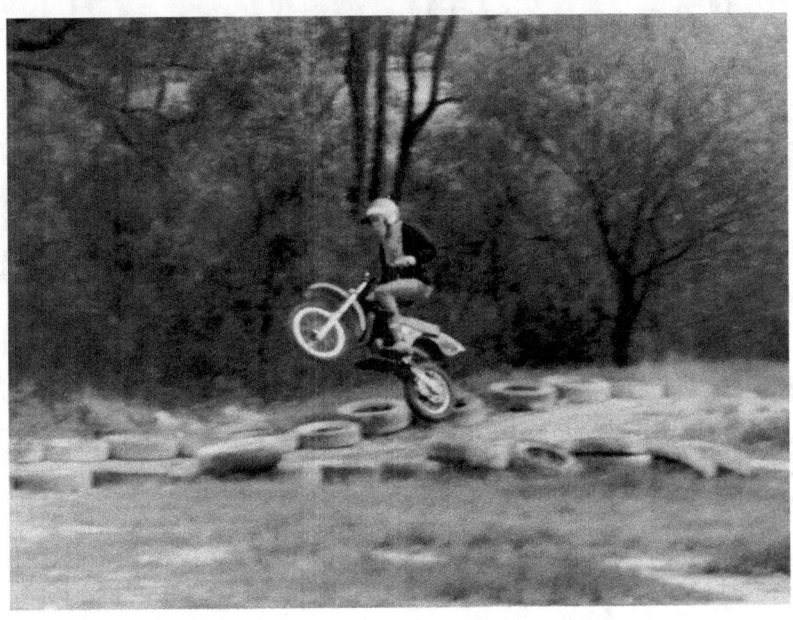

*This one didn't result in injuries.*

That was back at a time when protective gear wasn't such a big deal. We wore helmets, but body protection usually consisted of a jumper, jeans, gloves and boots.

Over a period of years, I worked my way up from the lower ranks to A grade. Along the way, I took part in the club's regular competitions. As well as the gymkhana riding, we competed in trials on small motocross bikes. There was also a "race" where you had to ride as *slowly* as possible between two marker tapes that were only 300mm apart—the last rider past the post took the prize. That certainly required some skill!

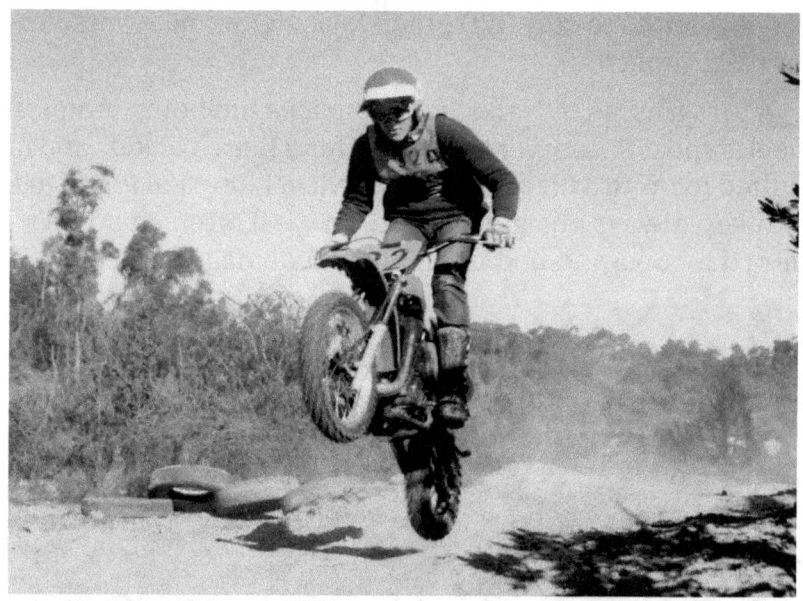

*I slowly moved up the club ranks.*

Finally, at the age of 17, I won the annual competition and was named number one rider in the club. I can still remember what a big honour that was and how amazing it felt to receive it. Everyone wanted that award.

I firmly believe that learning a skill and becoming good at it—no matter what it is—helps to set you up for success later in life.

## 1 | The lure of two wheels

*Leader of the pack*

As well as its rider training sessions, the Police Citizens Youth Club had a motorbike display team attached to it. I joined the team when I was about 11.

We were a group of 36 kids, ranging in age from eight or ten to 18, and we'd travel around to all the state and regional shows and perform precision riding and stunts.

When I joined the team, I was still a D grade rider and spent most of my time on the bench watching the other riders perform. I really wanted a chance to get out there and show what I could do.

I spent so much time as team reserve that I quit out of frustration, feeling like I wasn't being given a go. My mother was very supportive, telling me not to quit. "Keep persevering and you'll get a proper run," she'd say. Six months later, she convinced me to join back up again.

That was a good lesson in not giving up. Next thing I was back on the team, although still on the reserve bench.

I built up some more skill and eventually had enough practice to get to C grade, so they put me on the tail end of the display team.

It was an incredible experience for a kid; we were really putting on a proper display. We'd go to the Royal Easter Show in Sydney and we got to travel to New Zealand and Tasmania for their big annual shows as well as lots of country towns and regions.

We were the forerunner to the current display teams—

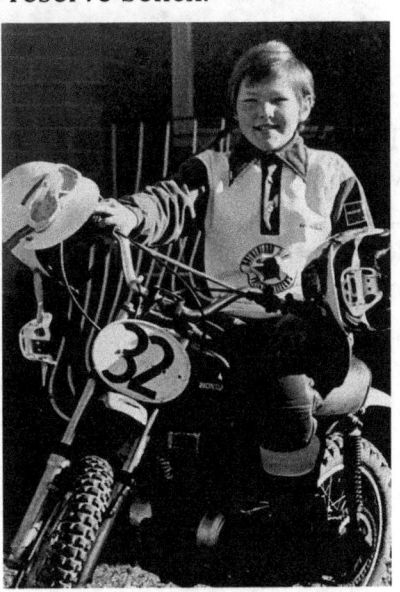

*Early years in the Precision Riding Team.*

motorbikes and cars—that put on shows at these big events now.

It was a real honour to be part of these shows; to be in the ring at the Royal Easter Show and hear the announcer say, "Here comes the Precision Riding Team! Thirty-six riders on motorcycles putting on the display!"

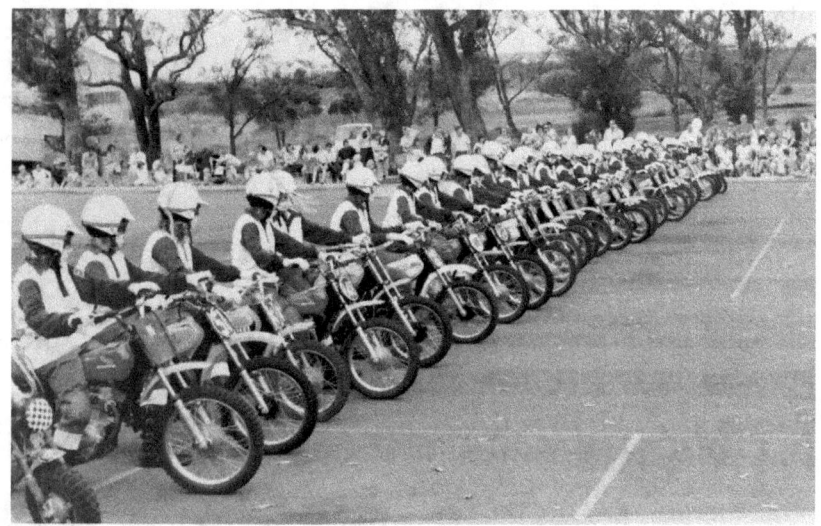

*Our team, ready for action*

There would be bursts of applause as we performed our routine, with the announcer describing our moves to the crowd. We'd do a crossover or jump and the audience would cheer. The kids in the crowd were in awe of what we were doing on these motorbikes.

Little by little, I worked my way from the back end of the team. I was consistent with my training and always turned up to the team practice sessions and the shows themselves. I learned something new every time.

Eventually I got the tap on the shoulder to say, "Mike, you're in line to be leader of this team if you're able to step up and take on that responsibility".

For someone who'd done their share of time at the bottom of the heap, that seemed incredible. I could barely believe I was being considered for such a role.

Over the next 12 months I worked as hard as I could to learn all the routines forwards and backwards. I could do them blindfolded! I practised, practised and practised until I got that official shoulder tap to be the leader of the display team.

Looking back, it was a big responsibility for a teenager. We had riders of all abilities in the team and every one of them needed lots of encouragement. I had to help them learn not only riding skills but also the routines and timing to make sure we got the precision right. The actual name of the team was "The Precision Riding Team", so there was pressure to do it perfectly.

We had to rehearse every element—movement, speed, direction—to be able to give a great performance without any mishaps—although accidents certainly happened!

Once, when I was leading the team, I slid into the fence that separated the arena from the spectators and nearly landed in the lap of a kid watching. I remember his eyeballs were the size of dinner plates. Somehow, I managed to stay on the bike, even though I'd crushed my ankle, and we finished the show.

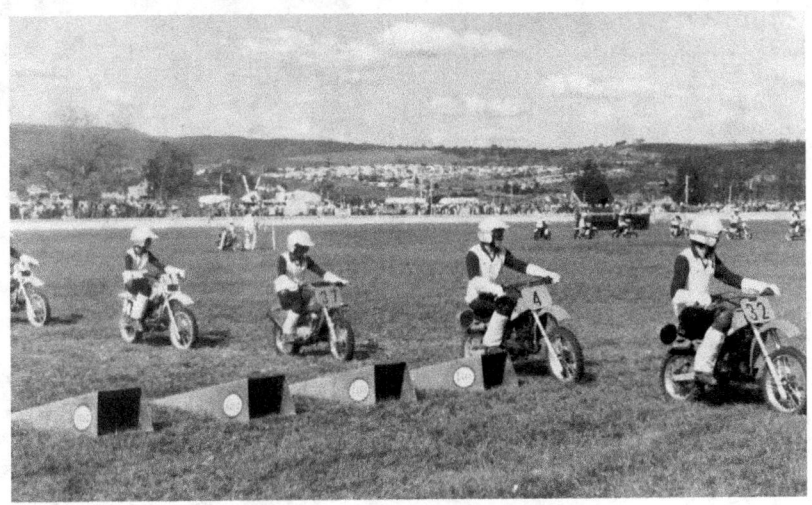

*Leading the way during a show*

As leader of the team, I had some official duties. There were times I was called on to go and meet the head of the Easter Show and say things like, "We're honoured to be here, and hopefully we can put on a good show for you."

At the end of our displays, we'd be mobbed by kids wanting to talk to us about riding motorbikes, because it was such a cool thing to do. It really was an amazing group to be a part of.

### The support squad

Of course, I didn't achieve all this alone, but as a child you take most things for granted. I had incredible support from my parents.

Dad didn't particularly like bikes and wasn't keen on us riding, but that was what we wanted to do, so he helped us get involved. The bike riding kept us occupied and out of trouble, and he could see the club had good influences on my life.

Dad worked extra jobs to earn the money to buy our various bikes over the years.

Mum was the one who took us to most of the events and training sessions, as Dad was often working. She became an expert at hooking up the trailer and helping us load the bikes on it. Mum was the glue that held our family together.

My Dad, an Irishman, has exceptional abilities—so ahead of his time in many ways.

He came from Ireland with nothing and created an extraordinary life for our family. He met Mum when she was 22 and travelling around the world, and followed her back to Australia.

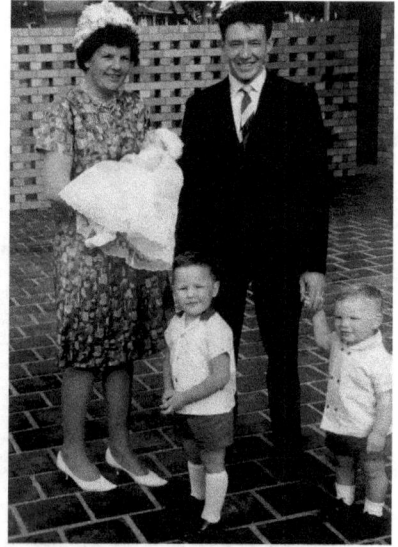

*My family, 1960s style. That's me in the middle.*

## 1 | The lure of two wheels

Dad was a living definition of working hard but there was never a complaint about it. He had made the decision that he would pay off his house and give his family a great life, and that's exactly what he did.

He never had time for illness, injury or anything that would stop him bringing home the bacon. He was on permanent night shifts and worked two other part-time jobs, so he often worked 16-hour days.

As we became teenagers, Dad recognised he needed to cut back some of his work hours to give Mum more support at home, so he quit his multiple jobs and went to teachers college to become a school teacher.

His phenomenal intellect meant he often ended up in feisty debates with lecturers about teaching methods and the correct answers in exams or assignments.

I can remember one occasion when Dad came home with the palms of his hands cut. It turned out these cuts were from his own fingernails digging into his hands during the lecture. Dad believed the lecturer was giving completely wrong information but he felt powerless to say anything, so he clenched his fist so tightly his nails cut into his flesh.

Despite numerous disagreements on various subjects, he became friends with many of his lecturers.

He finished college and took up teaching, but money was tight. Eventually he left teaching to take a job in a coal mine. He got badly injured in the mine but didn't stop working because we needed his bonuses to cover the mortgage—and our expensive motorcycle habit.

Dad went back to teaching and became a highly regarded high school educator. He taught all subjects across the curriculum from industrial arts to languages, maths, English, history, geography and everything in between. He was an incessant reader and would devour books on any subject.

I reckon Dad has done the equivalent of multiple university degrees, just through his own reading and research. I remember friends and relatives coming to him and saying, "Oh Sean, I've got an assignment, can you help me?" It might have been engineering, physics, language, nursing or any subject—it didn't matter to Dad. He would speak to the person to get a bit of background, then say, "Bring over a bottle of Scotch and I'll do the research—what mark would you like to get on your assignment? Do you need a pass? Do you need a high distinction?" And he would tailor the assignment to get whatever mark was needed.

He also got into running and decided he wanted to do a marathon. So, with three months of training and an altered diet, he completed his first marathon. He became a strong competitor with the local running club.

As a child, it was difficult to compete with Dad's considerable athletic and intellectual abilities. He was so good I could never run or train with him. When he ran, I couldn't even keep up with him—let alone beat him—on my pushbike.

I've often joked that Dad must have been one of the kids at school you love to hate, as he could do anything, mentally and physically, with no apparent effort.

He was also very good with his hands and could build almost anything, including detailed cabinetry and extensions to our house.

For Dad, all of this prowess was just normal. There didn't appear to be any work involved, he believed "it's just what you did". If you wanted a good mark, you got a good mark. If you wanted to run a marathon, you just did it.

I've since discovered, of course, that this is not the norm. Most people need to work hard to pass exams or get a good mark in an assignment. It's not uncommon for someone to train for years before they can run a marathon. It takes time to build the resilience, strength and endurance to be able to complete such an event—but that's not the philosophy I grew up with.

As a child and teenager, I observed from Dad's various accomplishments that all a person needed to achieve anything was to simply make a decision to do it. It appeared to me that once Dad decided he was going to do something, that was the end of it. He just made the decision and did it.

People would ask Dad, "Can you do such-and-such?" and he would say, "I'm sure I could but I've never tried."

When I was a kid, we had a home gym—which was unheard of at the time—because Dad believed physical strength was all-important. He was always the strongest guy in the room and continually challenged us kids to test our strength.

When most of my friends got pocket money for taking the bins out or doing the dishes, my siblings and I got it from doing chin-ups and push-ups. I was this lanky, skinny kid with such poor athletic ability I couldn't run out of sight on a dark night—but I always tried hard for Dad. In fact, once I did so many push-ups to try to impress him that I burst all the blood vessels in my neck. My neck was one giant scab for weeks!

I didn't know it back then but it turns out I was coeliac, which meant I didn't absorb all the nutrients from my food so I struggled to develop muscle. To Dad, I was just a scrawny kid who needed to toughen up.

I have to confess, Dad did most of my assignments at school. I'd leave them until the night before they were due, and he would do them overnight. I'd write them out in the morning in my handwriting and submit them.

I got by at school, but Mum and Dad encouraged me to leave after Year 10 and take an apprenticeship. A friend of a friend of Dad's had an opening for an electrical apprentice, so next thing you know, I'm on the path to becoming an electrician.

While I finished my trade I never felt particularly good at it, but it set me on the road to an incredible business later in life.

I'm eternally grateful for every sacrifice both my parents made to give us every opportunity to succeed.

And for the belief they instilled in me; that I could do *anything* I set my mind to.

# Adventures on dirt

**Mike**
*Riding professionally*

After finishing my electrical trade, I joined the police force. While I never really took to being a police officer on the beat, an amazing opportunity opened up. Very early in my time on the force, I was able to transfer to the driver training school at the Goulburn Police Academy where I became a motorcycle and car driving instructor.

I was the youngest instructor in the Academy's history. My experience with the Police Citizens Youth Club was so extensive it helped me get the role.

Of course, my fellow instructors at the Academy—some of them quite hard-bitten and all of them highly competitive riders—didn't exactly take kindly to this youngster joining their ranks. Some of them struggled to accept me and didn't bother hiding their feelings.

A month after I arrived at the Academy, they seized a chance to put me to the test. The local Goulburn motorbike club was hosting a competition. Many of the police instructors rode with the club, and there was also a healthy, competitive local riding community.

The event had three separate courses set up for C, B and expert riders. The expert course had challenges that were harder than anything I'd seen before. Competitors had to ride a bike over very difficult obstacles that included narrow planks and slippery conveyor belts set at various angles. They had to weave tight figure eights while bending over and picking up a 10 kilo sack of potatoes—crazy stuff!

It was a time trial, so you had to go as fast as you could—plus if you fell off or put your foot down at any time over the course, you were immediately disqualified.

The finale was that entrants had to ride over the top of a Volkswagen Beetle into a pile of loose car tyres and emerge out the other side without coming off the bike.

Another element that added to the challenge was that everyone in the expert category had to ride the same motorbike. You didn't get to practise on it, you just had to jump on it and go.

While I was busy gawking at the course and marvelling at its degree of difficulty, my colleagues entered me into the expert section, pitting me against the elite of the local bike club riders and the best of the Academy's riding instructors. Talk about being set up to fail!

I was scared, that's for sure. I'd never seen the locals ride. I didn't know what my competition was like. I was worried about riding a bike I'd never seen before, let alone practised on. I was also very concerned about my credibility if I didn't get through. My anxiety levels weren't helped as I watched other riders try the course while I waited my turn. Plenty of them fell off, hurt themselves or were otherwise disqualified.

The expert competition was held over two rounds; anyone not disqualified after Round 1 got to fight it out for the final prize in Round 2.

I remember riding onto the course and tackling the narrow plank, which is incredibly difficult at the best of times let alone on a foreign bike with 200 people watching. Everyone wanted to see the expert riders.

I navigated the bump at the end of the plank and went straight into the figure eights while having to lean over to pick up the sack of potatoes. That meant finishing the figure eights one-handed, with no access to the clutch because I was holding the accelerator in one hand and balancing the spuds in the other. The rest of the course is a blur, but I got through it cleanly.

The first time through, most of the riders were knocked out. Only five were left for the second round, including me. This only ramped up the pressure to new heights.

Added to that, there was another challenge. By the time we got to the second round, so many people had fallen off the bike it was in a sorry state of repair with twisted handlebars and bent brake and gear levers.

The course was exactly the same for Round 2 and I was placed in the middle of the pack. I watched two riders go ahead of me.

The crowd was eerily silent as they tackled each of the obstacles, then broke into wild cheering if they got through a section cleanly.

Both riders put their foot down during the course, which meant they were eliminated.

I felt a huge amount of pressure as I took my turn. All those years of practice kicked into gear; the drills and trials riding I'd completed with the Police Citizens Youth Club.

I managed to get through the course cleanly without falling off or putting a foot down.

Of the final two riders, one fell off and the other put his foot down. I was the only one who completed the course successfully.

*Disrupt Your Life*

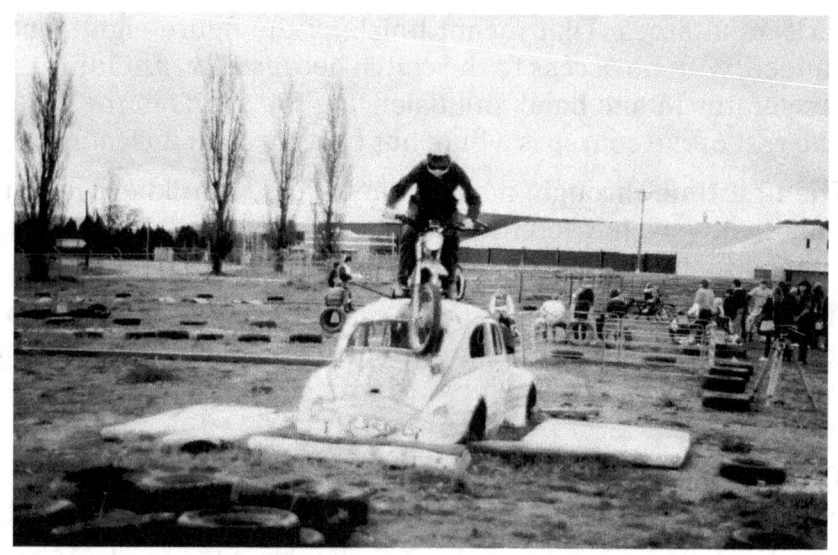

*That last VW obsctacle was a killer.*

The other riding instructors couldn't believe I was able to do it, especially those who had competed against me in the expert category. It was incomprehensible that I'd been able to beat not only them, but the local riders with their experience of the course. The locals certainly weren't happy about it; who was this blow-in who had arrived out of nowhere and shown them all up? A few egos were dented that day.

As the Academy's youngest instructor, this was the best thing that could have happened to me. It gave me immense credibility throughout my days as an instructor. My colleagues changed their attitude towards me as I had earned their respect. I felt a little begrudging in accepting their newfound friendship at first; after all, they had been having a go at me by entering me in the expert section without my knowledge, expecting me to fail. Still, I'd come through with the goods.

I settled into my job at the Academy and enjoyed the fact that I was now a professional rider. Because I had done so much riding on dirt at the Police Citizens Youth Club, part of my role involved teaching some of the newer motorcycle instructors how to ride off-road; handling rough and slippery surfaces, riding over logs, through creeks, over jumps, up rocky hills and down long, steep descents. I had been doing this type of riding for so many years, it came naturally to me.

In turn, I got expert instruction in road riding. This led to exhilarating experiences like riding the biggest BMW motorbikes in existence at race-level speeds around a tight track and then out on the open road. I can remember leaning the police bike over so far that I ground away the sirens and pannier boxes mounted on either side of the bike.

I became an all-round expert, skilled on both the road and the dirt. My time as a professional rider with the police built on the experience I'd gained throughout my childhood and teenage years. This set me up for the various rides I did later when I joined a motorbike club.

I didn't think about it too deeply at the time; it was all just riding. I never considered I was better than other riders—in fact I admired many of them.

As well as teaching motorcyle skills, I was also a police driving instructor. This involved a whole different level of patience: sitting in the passenger seat and giving instructions on how to accelerate very quickly, go around corners at high speed and handle a car in urgent response situations.

The lessons generally went without a hitch, but you have to remember my students were mostly testosterone-fuelled young men. Some wouldn't listen or didn't understand my instructions.

On one memorable occasion, a student skidded the car off the track at very high speed and we spun around three times.

When we came to a stop, our teeth still rattling, I had to be a model of patience. From the passenger seat, I calmly asked the student, "Now what do you think you've done wrong there?" as the dust continued to fly around the car.

This completely contradicted my genuine feeling, which was wanting to scream and punch the guy in the face for being such an idiot.

*A whole way of life*

I loved everything about bikes; I've often said that riding in the bush is the closest thing I've experienced to meditation because you have to be completely present and focused on that one thing, without any wandering of the mind.

My experiences as a child and teenage rider prepared me for many amazing years on bikes. As an adult, I joined a motorbike club and the people I rode with became my dearest friends.

As a member of the Clubman Tourers Motorcycle Club, I spent every spare moment riding with my mates on highways, back roads and dirt; away for weekends camping in the bush or staying in country pubs. Our love of the sport meant we shared similar values.

On a ride, we would automatically look out for each other; it was an understanding that never had to be put into words.

As we set out, we'd be looking at each other and doing a mental checklist: "Yep, they've got their helmet, they've got their gloves, their boots, they're prepared. They know how to repair a bike and are willing to do it if needed. They'll look out for me if I fall off and they can do first aid. We can help each other out in every way."

I guess what I loved was the sense of *community* in the club. Whether we were riding, socialising or helping each other move house, it felt like we were part of something special.

## 2 | Adventures on dirt

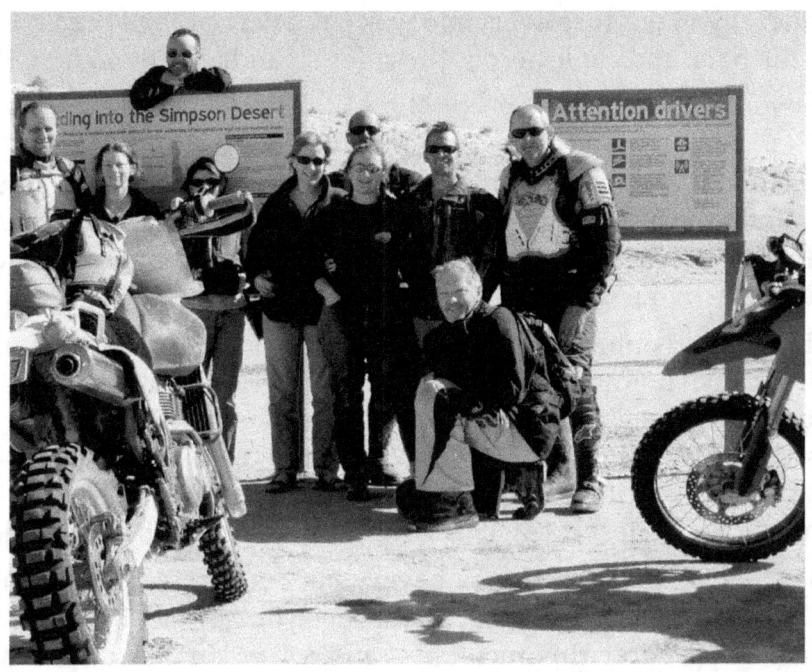

*The Clubman Tourers Motorcycle Club became a huge part of my life.*

There were times when new people would join our group and it didn't work out so well. That just highlighted the strength of the bond between us. That wasn't to say we didn't welcome newcomers; we did, as long as they shared the values that were important to us.

On one of our big rides in the Australian desert we had a new guy join us, a good mate of one of the others on the trip. We were told he was a competent rider, but he fell off a couple of times. The riding conditions were difficult, and he kept relying on others in the group to help him pick up his bike if he dropped it. If something needed repair, he didn't have the ability to fix it.

At the end of one of the big days out during the trip, this newcomer's mate ran out of fuel, 40 kilometres from Birdsville.

The new bloke rode to Birdsville to get petrol and he was supposed to ride back to help his stranded mate. That day, I was what we called "tail-end Charlie", the rider designated to check on anyone who had stopped, help do any repairs and generally make sure everyone was OK. I was riding at the back of the pack and came across the rider stranded with no fuel. He said, "I'm OK, my mate's gone into town to get petrol and he'll be back soon."

Based on that advice, I continued on into Birdsville. Who should I see but this newcomer fellow, wandering around town in a pair of shorts and a T-shirt, with absolutely no intention of going back to pick up his mate or give him fuel.

That responsibility then fell on my shoulders; I had to fill up a jerry can of fuel and take it to the stranded rider. But my day had been the biggest of the group because I'd been riding back and forth between everyone, stopping to help those who needed it. I was exhausted, and I now had to ride another 40 kilometres in the dark on a desert track, and 40 more kilometres back again.

I learned on that ride that not everyone's values were the same. When you're out in difficult conditions you have to look out for each other. After this incident—and a few smaller ones—we decided to tell the ring-in he wasn't welcome on the ride and couldn't stay with us in the group.

Those situations were rare. The great experiences far outweighed anything else. As riders, we got to explore places most people wouldn't visit, and we could do it in a relatively short time.

On one epic trip with my best mate, Reg, we criss-crossed the rugged northern deserts between Queensland and Western Australia.

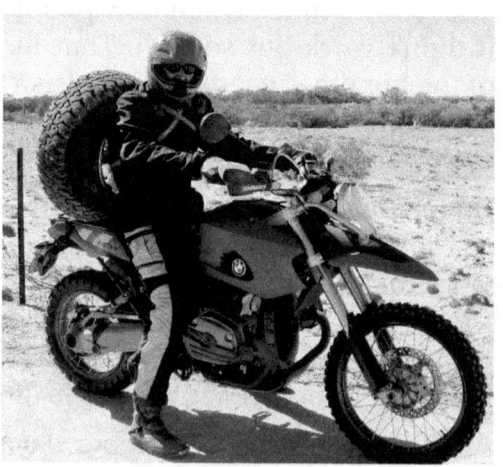

*Here I am in the Simpson Desert, rescuing a four-wheel drive that had a shredded tyre.*

That ride had it all: navigating corrugated sand tracks through desolate terrain with only sparsely-marked maps as our guide, experiencing remote townships and calculating our fuel levels in between stops.

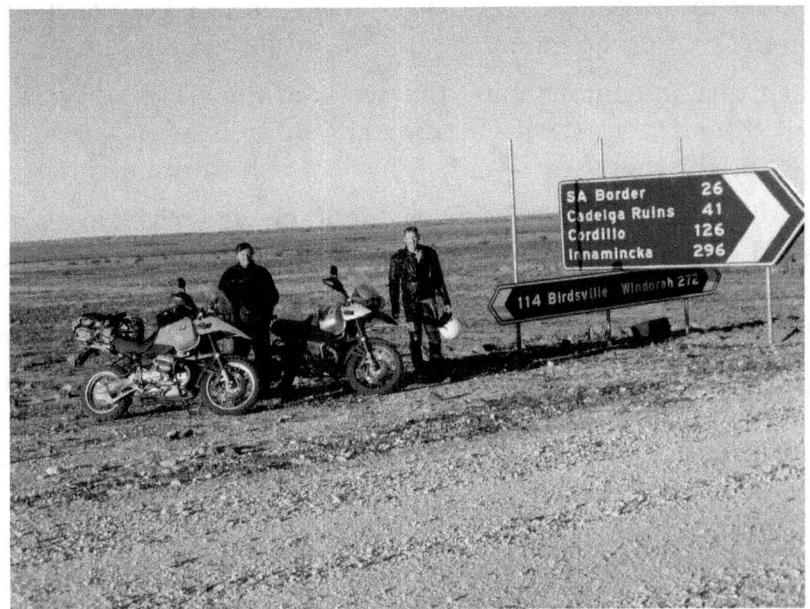

*Reg and I on one of our desert adventures*

We rode across the Donohue Highway, an outback track through the foothills of the Simpson Desert in Queensland, towards Alice Springs. Our next fuel, food and camping stop was meant to be a small Aboriginal settlement called Yuendumu, about 300 kilometres to the north-west.

You've probably seen one of those movies when a stranger arrives in a remote town and every local—down to the scrawny dog—stops, stares and snarls. These locals were less welcoming than that. We felt the urgent need to fuel up as quickly as we could and get out of there.

That meant we had to travel an extra 300 kilometres beyond our expected ride for the day to the next place with any kind of supplies, Rabbit Flat. We'd done our research and knew the location only had one service station/general store, which opened on Tuesdays from 9 am.

We set up one of our more interesting campsites of the trip out the front of the service station with 15 locals, all waiting it out for fuel and supplies. There was no aggression, but we clearly weren't part of the mix.

After that uncomfortable stop we continued riding west to Halls Creek in Western Australia and on to Lake Argyle in the Kimberley, where we went fishing for freshwater barramundi.

Heading back into the Northern Territory, we arrived at a place called Timber Creek and set up camp beside the picturesque river. It felt great to jump into the water after such a hot and dusty ride.

We enjoyed cooling off so much we ended up walking into the nearby pub still damp from our swim. The publican looked at us in horror. "You can't swim in there," he spluttered, "it's full of crocodiles!"

We learned he was right. We'd set up our tents in a croc haven. The only reason we didn't end up on their dinner menu was that, at the time we were in the water, they had all gone further down the river where there was a scheduled feeding time for the benefit of tourists. Needless to say, swimming was off the agenda after that.

From Central Australia we headed south to the Flinders Ranges, then to Adelaide. We took the Great Ocean Road to Melbourne and the New South Wales coast road for the homeward leg to Sydney.

We did that 10,000-kilometre trip, mostly on dirt tracks, in ten days including sightseeing. If you were to do it in any brand of car, you would need to allow at least a month to cover similar ground.

Of course, there were risks. Part of the riding took us along the Ghan rail track, and Reg found he couldn't handle such rough terrain. We split up for what was meant to be 24 hours. Reg was carrying some of our shared tools and I had the rest.

As luck would have it, I had a rail spike go through my back tyre at 120 km/h, so the tyre blew out very suddenly. I didn't crash, but when I stopped and checked out the damage, it turned out to be much more than a puncture repair.

The rail spike was so big it blew a hole in the tyre. I struggled to fix it on my own. I had some spare rubber to line the inside of the tyre, but Reg had the pump.

I was stuck on the rail track with no way of inflating the tyre. I couldn't go anywhere. I had a tent, water and a couple of muesli bars.

After a few uncomfortable hours, a four-wheel drive turned up, and the driver had a pump. I was able to get going and met up with Reg at William Creek eight hours later.

Looking back, I can see that riding motorbikes through the bush at high speed and having brittle bones as a result of coeliac disease is not a great combination. The trouble was, my coeliac condition wasn't diagnosed during my many years of riding.

There were plenty of spills—and for me, that meant plenty of broken bones.

On another desert adventure, I had to ride 2,000 kilometres home while only being able to use one arm after coming off the bike. The injured hand was the one I needed for the clutch, so I had to be inventive just to get the bike going.

I had to sit on the bike and push it forward with my toes. Once it got moving I slammed it into gear so the bike lurched forward, which was incredibly painful. I was then mobile and things were relatively easy as long as I didn't have to stop—or take a full breath.

When I finally got to hospital they found I'd broken my scapula, dislocated my shoulder, cracked my collarbone and fractured four ribs.

The thing was, I had a very strong and specific determination to get home from that ride, and I wasn't prepared to waste any time seeking medical attention.

Reg was meant to join me on that trip. We were avid adventurers together, having ridden all over Australia. I loved him like a brother. But Reg didn't feel he had enough experience to handle the harsh conditions of this ride, so he stayed home.

After my accident—while still out in the middle of nowhere, injured—I get a call from a friend telling me that Reg had been out riding to visit his mother in central western New South Wales and had also come off his bike.

Reg wasn't as lucky as me. Alone in the desert, I had to hear the news that my best friend had died.

That pain was far worse than any broken bones. All I wanted to do was get home so I could share my grief with our friends.

Did I ever consider the sport would nearly kill me?

Like any teenager, I never believed it would happen to me. As a young male, I didn't ever take those risks into account. I couldn't picture anything that was going to happen past the age of 20. When I was growing up, the term commonly given to motorcyclists was "temporary Australians", but I disregarded that notion completely.

I probably felt I had better training than the average motorbike rider, and maybe that was true.

It's hard to imagine what my 17-year-old self would have thought if he knew back then that at some point in his life he'd never be able to ride again.

# Coming to a sudden stop

*March 2010*
**Neryl**

Have you ever had one of *those* phone messages? The kind that make time stand still?

I received mine on a sunny Saturday afternoon. It was long enough ago that I still had a landline phone at home, but I rarely used it. It was even more rare for me to check for messages on it.

I'd been out for lunch with a girlfriend and was just getting home. As I opened the door of my apartment, I had a strange feeling that a message had been left on my landline. This made no sense, as anyone who knew me would first try calling my mobile and I'd had no missed calls in the last few hours. But as I passed through the lounge room, I looked at my home phone and noticed a light was flashing. There was, indeed, a message on it.

The voice on the recording belonged to Mike's mate, Matt, a giant of a bloke whose colourful turn of phrase came from his knockabout upbringing in country New South Wales. The two of them were in a group that had gone motorbike riding early that morning in the bush near Nowra, south of where we lived in Wollongong.

The message began, "Mike's had a bit of an accident…"

My first thought was, what does "bit of an accident" mean this time? Mike and I had only been together for about 18 months, and in that time I'd heard plenty of stories about crashes and near-misses as part of his long-held love of motorbikes. Only recently he'd had a relatively serious spill on the bike that put him in hospital with broken ribs.

There was often teasing around the dinner table when his three kids, Briana, Connor and Abby, recited the injuries Mike had sustained each year since they'd been born.

Matt's message, in a monotone devoid of emotion, went on to say, "He's broken both his legs. He's being airlifted to St George Hospital."

That sounded a whole lot more serious. Both legs? Airlifted? I'd been a television journalist long enough to know they didn't put you in a helicopter and fly you to hospital for no reason. *Two* broken legs? I couldn't begin to fathom how someone as active as Mike would cope with that. And St George Hospital? A major trauma centre.

"Mike's had a bit of an accident. He's broken both his legs. He's being airlifted to St George Hospital." Three sentences signalling the end of our current life, the start of a new and uncertain one.

I had a sudden sensation of my world screeching to a halt.

My first thought was, *get in the car, drive the one and a half hours to the hospital, and do it now!* The problem was, there was no car. On my way back from lunch, I'd left it at the car wash a block from my house and was planning on collecting it later.

I sprinted back to the car wash, a million confused thoughts colliding in my head. I was met with a scene of high farce, which seemed to play out in slow motion in direct contrast to my escalating panic. They wouldn't give me back my car.

"It's not finished!", the young car wash attendant argued, stubbornly wielding a soapy sponge at my half-clean vehicle. "I don't care!", I snapped back. Explaining the situation only seemed to make him more determined to present me with the cleanest car that had ever come out of their facility.

After further cajoling he reluctantly handed me the keys, casting a sorrowful eye at the car's unwashed rear panels.

Finally, I was driving up the freeway to Sydney. The phone ran hot as I called Mike's family to let them know what I knew—which wasn't a lot. I tried to find out more from Matt but couldn't get hold of him.

It's interesting what goes through your mind when you're in a situation like that. It's like being in the centre of a vortex; the rest of the world is going about its Saturday-afternoon business and you're acting from a place of single-minded focus based on one piece of information.

I rang the hospital from the car and was surprised that, for a medical facility as large as St George, the person who answered the phone knew a critically injured patient was coming in by helicopter. She was relieved I had called because they had no other information about the patient. I was able to provide a few personal details.

I gathered the helicopter was still airborne at that stage; it must have been almost overhead as I stood in my apartment listening to that message from Matt.

I found out later Matt had retrieved Mike's mobile phone and had gone through it for names and numbers he recognised. When he saw my name, he called the first number that appeared, which happened to be my home phone.

If I wasn't anxious enough as I scooted up the freeway, there was another reason the dash to St George Hospital was filling me with dread. It was probably my least favourite place in the world. Many years before, at the age of 17, I had a major spinal operation for a condition called *scoliosis*, a sideways curve of the spine that can have serious consequences. Royal-watchers will recognise it as the same condition suffered by Princess Eugenie, who now actively raises awareness of scoliosis and promotes its early identification.

My operation involved having a 9" steel rod grafted to my spine using bone taken from my hip. Afterwards, I was in a full plaster body cast for six months—no showers that entire time.

As a result of that experience, I couldn't stand the smell of a hospital ward. In fact, when I became a TV reporter, I put up my hand to do medical stories so I'd be forced to go into hospitals. I wanted to teach myself to overcome my fear.

Over time, that made a difference. But here I was, driving to a hospital where I expected to find Mike badly injured—just *how* badly I didn't yet know. And it wasn't just any hospital; it was *the* hospital where I had my spinal operation.

Finally I got there, and by this time it was early Saturday evening. If you've had the misfortune of being in an emergency waiting room on a Saturday night in Sydney—or any capital city, for that matter—you'll know what a crazy and confusing scene it is.

When I told the receptionist who I was, she ushered me through a door immediately. Normally such prompt service would be welcome, but this didn't feel in any way good. Mike's brother, John, was already there. He'd had no news of Mike's condition.

We were taken to a colourless, minimally furnished room, somewhere in the back of the emergency department.

As I sat, I remembered the sight of Mike leaving my apartment early that morning in his riding gear. The image was so vivid, and I couldn't get it out of my mind. I wondered how different he would look the next time I saw him—if I got to see him.

The long wait began.

## Mike

I'd had a huge week leading up to that Saturday. As the owner and sole technician of a fibre optics business, I spent plenty of time on the tools as well as trying to juggle the books, talk to customers and order supplies. I was in the middle of a huge project at a coal mine in the Hunter Valley, about three hours' drive from home, plus I'd been doing double shifts so I could

## 3 | Coming to a sudden stop

complete another big project in Sydney. The glamorous life of a small business owner.

I was totally shattered and could have slept for two days. But I'd also had a call from a group of mates I'd ridden motorbikes with all my life, and they wanted to go for a ride in the bush down the coast. One of my newer bike-riding friends, Matt, was joining us.

The decision to go riding with them was one of those life-defining choices that seem completely inconsequential at the time. While riding was my number one pastime—something I'd done since childhood, as I shared in the previous chapters—I had also been dabbling recently in another sport, surf ski paddling. It was a toss-up whether I went paddling or riding that day.

Living on the coast in Wollongong, the appeal of getting involved in an ocean sport was huge. In between the bike rides, I was learning to paddle a ski; it wasn't the exhilaration of hurtling through the bush at high speed on two wheels, but it had other charms. Paddling a long, skinny vessel kilometres out into the ocean puts you face to face with nature in a very immediate way. I was getting used to the regular encounters with dolphins, seals, sharks and even whales.

I stayed at Neryl's apartment on Friday night, with the ski on the roof of my car ready to go for a paddle. The invitation from my riding mates was also very much in my mind. Even though I was exhausted from the relentlessly busy week, I set the alarm to get up early, leaving the final choice until the morning.

In the end, I opted to take the ski off the roof, hook up the trailer with the dirt bike in it, and set off for a big day of riding.

Actually, it was more than just a ride. Even though by then I was in my forties, I was competing at a top level in cross-country Enduro riding. One of my goals was to compete in the Australian Safari, a mammoth race across the desert. Each time I went out with this group we were getting ready for the next big event.

It wasn't about going for a nice ride though the bush. This was proper race preparation; making sure we were fit and healthy, the bikes were prepared, we could handle pretty well any conditions.

Neryl often joked about how competitive and determined I was, but I never realised it. When I went out with the motorcycle club, sometimes with 30 or more on the ride, I would invariably ride at the front of the group. It's true that if anyone came up beside me, I nudged ahead and stayed in front. I wasn't trying to have a competition—that was just what I did.

After making the choice to ride that morning, I can remember only small glimpses of what followed. I have a vague recollection of heading down the coast to the spot where we'd go off-road for the day. There were six of us in the group.

I recall I had loaned one of my bikes to a mate from the bike club, Brendan, who was riding with us. He had a minor crash during the morning. While I wasn't worried about the small amount of damage to the bike, I remember him apologising to me.

One of the other guys with us also had an accident and while he wasn't hurt, he damaged his bike badly. I was the only one who had the equipment to get it going again.

I can recall helping him repair his bike, but that's the last thing in my memory of the entire ride. Someone took photos of me doing the bike repair and it was late morning. Seeing the photos prompts vague flashes of memory, but that's about it.

What happened from there? I only know what others have told me.

We were riding at high speed on a rugged section of trail; apparently one person was in front of me and four were behind.

When my mates got to the end of the track, I wasn't there.

For reasons still unknown, I was flung—along with my bike—far off the side of the track, so that when the four riders behind me came past, they saw nothing, not even dust. I must have been far enough ahead that the dust cleared before they arrived.

## 3 | Coming to a sudden stop

At the end of the trail, the whole group went back to look for me. They spotted my bike first, then saw me in the bush.

Apparently I was speaking, or at least making noises. I was lying on my back with both legs sticking out sideways at angles legs shouldn't be pointing at. My left femur was poking out through the back of my leg.

I have lots of ideas about what happened, but they're only theories. It appears I hit a stationary object while I was doing more than 100 kilometres an hour. That was never going to end well.

Whatever I hit remains a mystery. From the description of the accident location and the photos I've seen, there was no obvious cause. I came off the track on a ridge: a flat, fast riding area. The bike ended up in a better state than me.

Most damage was on the topside of the rear of the bike. Because there was no damage at the front, it seems I hit something soft and large, possibly a wild boar or kangaroo. It was soft enough that the impact was absorbed and didn't damage the bike. It was also heavy enough to cause me to fly forward, forcing the front of the bike down and sending the back wheel into the air.

That's the only theory that makes sense to me. Hitting a very large and heavy animal at high speed caused the bike to come to an abrupt stop. Strangely, there was no sign of any animal or injury to an animal.

Later, when I was semiconscious in hospital, I apparently insisted to Neryl that there'd been a four-wheel drive vehicle on the track. This made no sense and, according to the others on the ride, simply wasn't possible. In a separate conversation I insisted to another friend that I'd speared off the track after clipping a rock, then hit a fallen log.

Whatever the cause, on impact I slid up the petrol tank to where my legs hit the handle bars. The left leg snapped clean through the femur and my body then rotated around that broken leg, causing the right leg to shatter in a spiral. My body continued to fling forward, crushing five vertebrae in my spine to a point where fragments of bone smashed off and were stuck between my spine and lungs.

I hit my head and suffered a brain injury, which would result in amnesia. You can imagine there was significant other damage as well.

I must have completed a spectacular front roll. If I'd ever wanted to join the Crusty Demons high-risk performance team, now was my chance—but unfortunately I didn't have an audience to appreciate it.

My bike continued to somersault and landed tail-first on me—hence the damage to the rear of the bike.

I didn't sever my femoral arteries but there was so much damage to the legs that I lost a huge amount of blood. My thighs were blown up like balloons.

The riders with me were fantastic; they gave the GPS coordinates of our location to the ambulance control so a helicopter could come straight to us. Paramedics were also despatched by road. Some of my mates rode off the track to the nearest intersection and led the road ambulances in. Their actions probably saved my life.

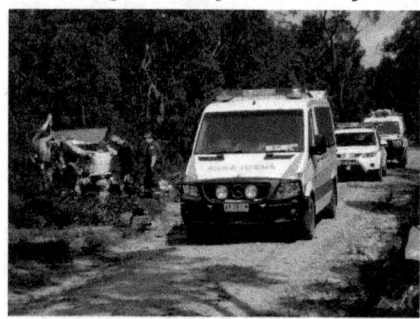 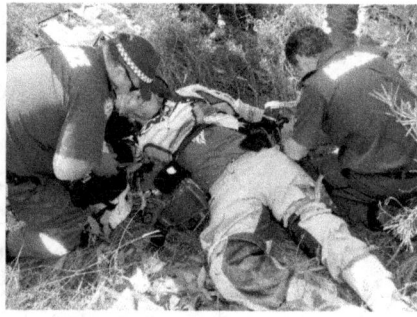

*Thanks to my mates, the paramedics got to me in the bush.*

At that stage there was apparently a good chance I wasn't going to make it. One of the guys took photos at the scene, and you can see the paramedics talking to my mates. They're telling them, "Look, we've done the best we can for Michael, but we don't think he's going to make it as far as St George Hospital."

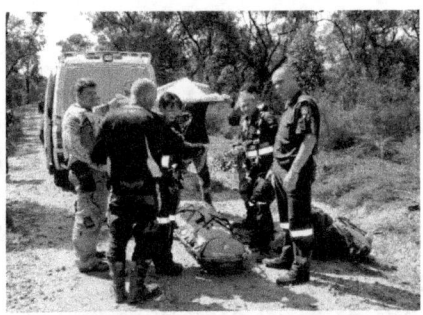

*"We've done our best for Michael..."*

It was incredible how fast the chopper got there. We were way out in the bush, and it was only because my riding mates—always looking out for me—had the presence of mind to give the precise GPS points that help arrived when it did.

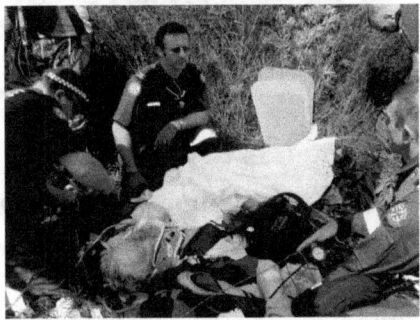

*Getting treatment before the airlift*

I was treated by the paramedics on the ground and given lots of what they call a "green whistle", a type of pain-killer. They did what they could to straighten my legs and put them in splints.

As the helicopter roared overhead, I was put on a stretcher and winched up, clouds of dust billowing around me.

I got the ride of my life—the best seat in the house—and I don't remember a thing.

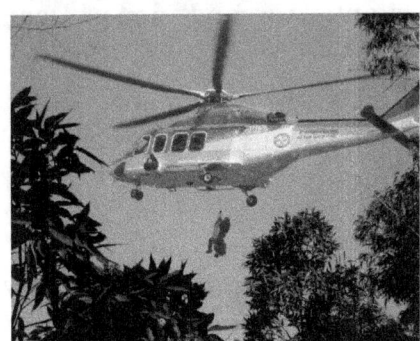

*Winching a crewman down to pick me up*

*Leaving only dust in my wake*

**Neryl**

The waiting dawdled on.

Sitting in that space, the "crying room" as I heard it described later, John and I could hear the pulsing and beeping of monitors and other equipment. At various times footsteps hurried past. Nearby, someone was sobbing.

At one point I went to go to the bathroom, and staff stopped me. One of the emergency department's regular weekend visitors was in the throes of a violent, drug induced frenzy and the area had gone into partial lockdown. It just added to the overall experience.

Seconds, minutes and hours dragged by. At some point I remember eating pizza; I have no idea where it came from.

We still didn't know what state Mike was in. I had no more information than when I got that phone message earlier in the day. I was making regular contact with Mike's parents in Queensland and his three kids, but there was nothing new to say. I felt numb and disconnected, and at the same time had a terrible fear about why there'd been no update in such a long time. I expected a sombre messenger in scrubs to suddenly appear in the doorway with the worst possible news, like on a TV show.

It was after midnight when a doctor did emerge. He was calm and quietly spoken, and he said we could see Mike. That was the first confirmation that Mike had survived.

The doctor led us through a now silent emergency department to a curtained cubicle—and there he was.

It's hard to describe how I was feeling in that moment. I was moving robotically, like none of this was real. The space we were led to was silent and dark and its centrepiece was an almost lifeless figure, lying very flat. It was a version of Mike, but not the person I knew. I felt unmistakeable relief that he was alive but I could barely breathe, not knowing what to expect next.

## 3 | Coming to a sudden stop

I had two first impressions as I gazed down at him. One, he looked very different from the tall, confident guy in motorbike leather striding out of my apartment that morning. Two, he was absolutely filthy, like he'd been caked in dark makeup.

At first I couldn't work out why, then it dawned on me. As he was being winched up into the helicopter, the downdraft had blown dirt and mud all over him.

He wasn't moving, but he did open his eyes. I tried to talk to him, but he couldn't seem to see or hear me. I felt like I had to whisper in the silence.

I leaned over, right in front of his face, in the hope of getting a sign of recognition. I was rewarded with a weak smile.

Isn't it amazing, when faced with that kind of situation, often our first response is to go into "busy mode"? When we're paralysed and helpless, we look for something practical to do.

I suddenly thought, "I have to clean him up!" and started searching the cubicle for something to use. All I could find was a roll of very coarse paper towel and cold water. John and I began scrubbing at Mike's face to get the dirt off.

He was vaguely conscious by now; he knew who I was and insisted he had to go back to the bush to the find big four-wheel drive he'd hit. He said this numerous times, but nothing else was coherent.

Our scrubbing was only partly successful. His face looked cleaner—very pale under the mud—but I remember feeling frustrated that I couldn't get the dirt from around his eyes. Lying broken on an emergency bed looking a little like some glam rock star seemed pretty incongruous.

The doctor came in and said, matter-of-factly, "He's going to have to be put in traction, and it could get a bit rough". I'll never forget this part.

The medical staff asked me to step outside the cubicle, and they pulled the curtain across. I didn't know what torture they were administering in there, but all I could hear were Mike's piercing screams.

To this day, that memory makes me feel sick. I have never felt as helpless as in that moment.

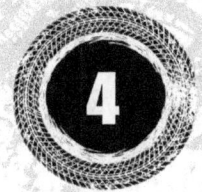

# Memories that are best forgotten

**Mike**

I have only tiny flickers of memory from that first night. Then again, I don't know if they're actual memories or whether I've been told about things that happened.

Because of the head injury and amnesia, I don't remember much of the entire week leading up to the accident and can only recall snippets of the whole hospital experience.

There's a vague shred of recollection about Neryl and John trying to clean my face. Neryl has told me about the screaming when I was put in traction—I'm grateful I don't remember that.

I have a distant memory of being in a room on my own, hooked up to what seemed like medieval torture instruments. Holes had been drilled into the sides of both my knees, and horseshoe-shaped pieces of metal had been inserted. Ropes were attached to these hooks, with weights on the end of the ropes to pull my legs straight and stretch my knees away from my hips.

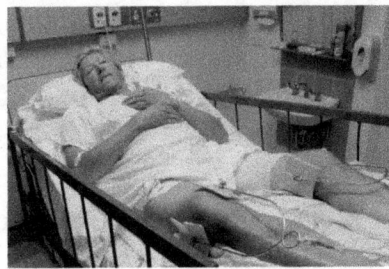
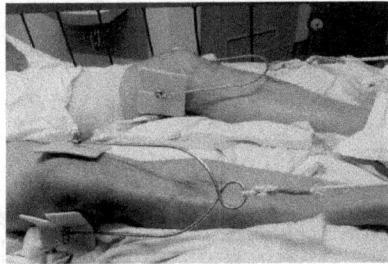

*I wasn't going anywhere in a hurry.*

The weights continually dragged me down the bed until my feet were pressing hard against the sharp edges of the rails at the foot of the bed. Every two hours the weights had to be lifted so I could be dragged back up the bed, which caused absolute agony. Despite the nursing staff having to do this and my family protesting, no solution was ever sought. It wasn't until I had left the hospital that a physiotherapist explained that the bed should have been set up on an angle to prevent me being dragged down by the weights.

My left leg had a clean break, straight across the bone. The right leg was much more of a mess; it had sustained a spiral fracture which meant the bone was shattered to smithereens. Fragments of bone had exploded throughout my thigh.

I know now that I also had multiple fractured vertebrae. The problem was, these injuries went undiagnosed throughout my entire hospital stay. Everyone was fixated on the damage to my legs and, to a lesser extent, my brain injury. Even after such a traumatic accident, I was never X-rayed for possible spinal injuries.

That seems incredible—believe me, it confounds me to this day—but I was in such a world of agony that I wasn't able to pinpoint the precise sources of pain at that time.

I know the pain was off the chart, even though I was off the planet on morphine-based medication. One minute I'd be conscious and high as a kite (apparently I said some very strange things that are better forgotten) and next minute I'd be comatose; I just couldn't keep my eyes open.

Now and then I'd have random flashes of insight like, "Oh, that's right, the surf ski is still on the roof of my car and it doesn't belong to me, I borrowed it; I'd better call the guy and let him know to pick it up!" Of course, the ski wasn't on the roof of my car; I'd made a fateful decision on that Saturday morning to remove it and go riding instead.

After four days of traction, I had surgery to insert titanium rods from the hip to the knee in both legs. These were meant to hold me up in place of my femurs, which were now useless.

In the lead-up to the operation, I remember telling the surgeon I had really long legs so he had to choose rods that were long enough to do the job. Those words came back to haunt me later.

## Neryl

It's amazing how quickly your life can change. Mike and I had certainly had some adventures in the relatively short time we'd been together. Those memories included camping in the dirt on a football oval at Condobolin in western New South Wales during a big bike competition, me singing a whole repertoire of songs into my helmet to quell my nerves as a pillion passenger on the back of Mike's bike and collecting Mike from a country hospital after one of his previous spills.

But this was a new level. Now I was keeping vigil as he lay hooked up to equipment, mostly not recognising me or even aware I was there.

It's hard to say why I threw myself into the role of carer so quickly; it's not that anyone asked it of me. My own hospital experience certainly played a part. While that had happened many years before, I still remembered the difference it made having people at my bedside when I was conscious.

I spent as much time as I could at the hospital. I took leave from my job and my days blended into a ritual of driving to and from the hospital and sitting at Mike's bedside. While I wanted to be there, another reason that compelled me to spend so much time in the ward was the very obvious lack of nursing and support staff.

The nurses at St George worked at absolute capacity; they provided the best care their limited time would allow, but they were clearly stretched to extraordinary lengths. It was apparent they relied heavily on patients' families to step in and fill the yawning care gap.

I was by no means an experienced caregiver, but I got into the groove of feeding, bathing and the teeth-cleaning routine that always marked the end of my evening visit.

It took me a while to get used to Mike's unpredictable behaviour as a result of the medication he was on. I remember coming in to see him after the first surgery to put rods in his legs, expecting him to be sound asleep. Instead, I found him sitting up in bed, resplendent in full hospital gown, with a laptop in front of him and a phone to his ear. He was giving very animated instructions to someone and presumably making decisions about the running of his business.

We've joked since that it was the most profitable year the company ever had. Actually, that's not true; it went on to be even more successful. There must have been some confused individuals on the other end of those medication-fuelled phone calls.

The nurses at St George came from diverse cultures and some spoke very little English. I came into Mike's room on one occasion to find a young Chinese nurse looking very confused. Mike was just waking up and she was asking him, "You have pen? You have pen?" He was getting agitated, but she asked him again. "You have pen?" This time he snapped at her, "Why would I have a f**king pen, I've just had an operation!"

I had to intervene and point out, "Mike, she's asking you if you have pain".

In those situations, you just have to laugh. Mike didn't see the funny side at the time, but that remains one of my favourite stories from the whole hospital experience.

A bit later in the hospital journey, when all the various tubes in Mike's body were removed, I got further confirmation—as if I needed it—that I never wanted a full-time career as a nurse. I got a taste of the pan room.

We used to joke that I should have been on the hospital payroll; it's a serious comment on our health system that there were so few staff on the ward they simply couldn't look after the patients' basic needs. If someone wanted a bed pan, often a visitor would have to go and fetch it.

I went into the pan room many times to collect an empty pan for Mike or one of his ward-mates, but I always said, "I'm not taking it back afterwards". You have to draw the line somewhere.

## Mike

There are patches of memory about visitors; I'm aware of waking up after surgery and seeing one of my bike club mates there. I was having a great conversation with him—I don't remember what I said, but I know he was surprised I was able to speak with such animation.

Apparently that was the conversation in which I described the accident in detail; glancing off a rock on the track and then hitting a fallen tree or log in the undergrowth beside the trail. This is all news to me, after the event. I told him the bike hit whatever it was and stopped dead, and that "I went straight through the (handle) bars standing up and nearly took my legs off." It sounds plausible but I have no memory of it now; and it's different to comments I made to other people when I was at various stages of grogginess. Who knows?

I have occasional flashes of Neryl being there, seeing my brother, John, and a couple of others from the bike club, including Brendan who was there on the day of the accident.

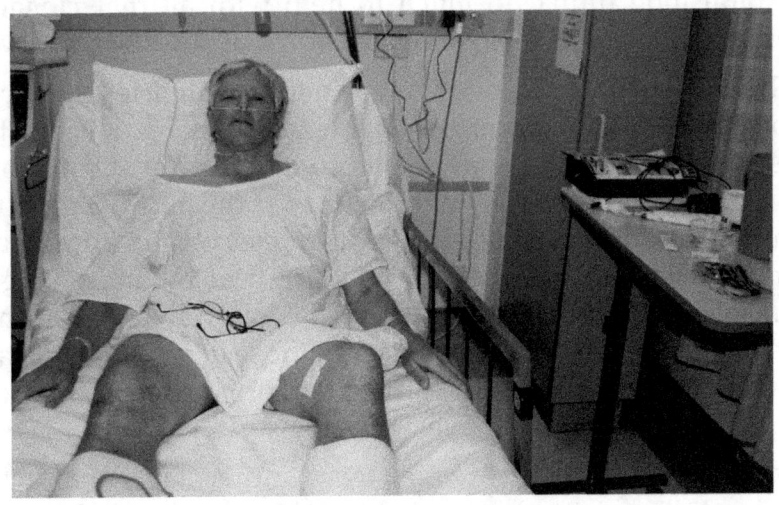

*Me with my patchy memory*

Not long after the surgery they moved me from the single room to a ward with three other people. Neryl tells me it was busy and noisy with little privacy for me. I'd get bathed or have my gown changed without anyone worrying too much about my modesty. Apparently a bit later in the piece they wheeled me to the toilet a couple of times and left the door wide open so everyone in the ward could see straight in. My care factor was nil, thanks to the medication. Probably a good thing.

Mum and Dad arrived from Queensland, and one thing I do vaguely recall (and Neryl takes great delight in reminding me) is greeting them in my loose, backless hospital gown with the words, "You're probably going to see a few things you haven't seen for a long time." That still raises a laugh.

I can't remember being able to eat much during those weeks, but at mealtimes the ward actually smelled great because many of the patients were ordering pizzas, Subway—you name it and it was delivered to our ward. That tells you more about the quality of the hospital food than any description I could provide.

I know that what they did feed me wasn't always the most appropriate. I experienced first-hand that strong pain and anti-inflammatory medications clog up the system—and the hospital food didn't do much to help with all that clogging. Here I was, trapped in hospital and stuck in other ways as well.

I also had a couple of other, more delicate, injuries. Picture a motorcycle with a person on it, then a sudden collision. The first thing that happens when you come to an abrupt stop on a bike is you slide forward up the seat, over the petrol tank to the handle bars. Everything—and I mean *everything*—that made contact with the petrol tank ended up bruised and enlarged. I have some memory of a very uncomfortable experience, getting checked over to make sure all those bits were intact and functioning, including a full ultrasound of my undercarriage. If that brings tears to your eyes, I apologise.

My three kids were young teenagers at this stage, and during their regular visits they'd run amok on the ward. They put some wheelchairs to really good use, racing each other around the place.

It was so great to have them there, even if I wasn't fully present. My eldest daughter, Briana, showed incredible strength and seemed to make friends with all the other patients around me in the ward. I'm told there was a fellow opposite me who was very ill with a terminal disease, and she propped herself up beside him and asked him, "What's wrong?" Far from feeling intruded upon, he loved the attention and told her his life story. She was wonderful not only in helping to look after me but talking to and caring for the other patients in the ward; helping them to feel good about themselves.

John was also a great supporter, and one day he decided I needed some fresh air. Ignoring Neryl's protests, he loaded me into a wheelchair (still clad only in my hospital gown) and wheeled me out of the hospital and around the block to a coffee shop. It was a windy day, and I think drivers waiting at the traffic lights got more than they bargained for when we crossed the street.

Because of my amnesia, there was concern about my brain injury and the possibility of permanent damage. I had to do daily memory tests, but I think the results were less than accurate thanks to well-meaning hospital occupational therapists.

A therapist would show me some cards, maybe half a dozen or a dozen at a time. Each had a different picture; a flower, pot plant, umbrella and so on. The next day they would return and ask, "Can you remember the cards we showed you yesterday?"

I'm sure I was supposed to remember them on my own, but I had little hope of doing that. I think the therapists didn't want me to feel embarrassed in front of my visitors in the ward because they would prompt me by saying things like, "Oh, Michael, what would you take if you were going out in the rain?"

I'd reply, "a raincoat" or something like that and they'd say, "No, no, something you might hold in your hand."

"Oh, umbrella!"

Then they'd ask, "What would you wear on your feet?"

"Oh...a boot."

So, I'd pass that particular test.

Those assessments weren't doing much to check the extent of my brain injury or amnesia, so other than some counselling later, I didn't have any direct treatment for my head trauma. And at this point, my back injuries were still undiagnosed.

I was feeling extreme discomfort in my back and staff felt enough concern to try out several types of mattresses in an attempt to help me sleep. Despite that, I was not examined for the possibility of spinal injuries.

Three weeks had passed since the crash. I didn't have a strong sense of the passing of time; the days blurred together. I was still so heavily medicated that I didn't comprehend—not for a long time—how badly damaged I was.

Staff started to raise the possibility of having me transferred from St George to Wollongong Hospital, closer to home. This was great news for Neryl and my family, who were making the regular three-hour round trip to care for me.

I vaguely remember being loaded by stretcher into an ambulance for the trip from St George to Wollongong. I wasn't allowed to travel any other way. I have an idea I was hooked up to two separate drips, presumably a pain-killer and something else.

It feels disloyal to criticise the public hospital in your own backyard, but I have to say my stay in Wollongong was the lowlight of all my treatment. By then, I was starting to become more aware of my surroundings. In many ways, I wish I could forget the pieces I remember so clearly.

The experiences and observations I'm about to describe were formally reported to health authorities, once we'd had a chance to let it all sink in. In response, we were told there was nothing further to investigate and no action would be taken. I make no apology for this next section reading like a "house of horrors" tale, as these were my direct experiences.

In any situation where vulnerable people are treated without dignity, respect and care, the facts need to be brought to light and appropriate action taken. I can only hope that, nearly a decade on, our society has evolved and we now treat these cases in a different way. I also hope things are very different at an operational level at that particular hospital.

I found myself in a four-person room, with an elderly woman in the bed diagonally opposite me. She was openly distraught about sharing a room with three males; I gather having mixed wards is normal these days but it doesn't give much regard to the feelings of the patients, particularly older people, who aren't used to being in such a vulnerable state in front of strangers of the opposite sex.

The nursing staff in that ward seemed to have a collective bad attitude, and patient care wasn't high on their priority list. One day I rang and rang my buzzer—I can't remember the reason but it must have been important. After a long delay, a nurse came in and told the four of us in the room, "It doesn't matter how many times you push that button, we will come when we're good and ready".

During the night, it was virtually impossible to get staff to bring bed pans and bottles for toilet use, so I had to use the same bottle repeatedly. My bottles were regularly overflowing and not emptied. On a number of occasions, full bottles that had been left beside my bed were kicked over by staff.

There never seemed to be any water available; unlike St George where it was served from the tap in plastic jugs, Wollongong only served bottled water. On more than one occasion Neryl had to go searching for water for me and received a sour response from staff when she asked for it.

One senior nurse, in particular, was downright nasty to some of the patients, including the poor woman in my room who seemed to suffer additional humiliating treatment. She was often left uncovered, with her nightgown open and curtains around her bed not properly closed, which was awkward for all concerned. She was frequently crying and upset.

One day—and Neryl also witnessed this incident—this nurse came in with another and told the woman opposite me she had to get out of bed and walk. The woman protested loudly that she couldn't stand up on her own.

Next thing, the nurses had the lady out of bed and were holding her up, one on either side. She was told to stand on her own, which caused her to cry hysterically. We were trying not to eavesdrop, which was impossible with only a curtain separating us from the scene, when we heard a sickening crash and saw the woman on the floor, sobbing. I didn't see the fall so I can't say for sure that the nurses let her go, but I certainly saw the results. She was chastised like a naughty child in front of everyone else in the room.

The man in the bed directly opposite me spoke no English and his relatives were disgusted by his poor treatment. When meals were delivered, staff would leave his food out of his reach and line of sight, so he was unaware it was there. Later, they would come and collect the full tray of food, without trying to ask why he hadn't eaten anything or communicate with him in any way. When his family visited, he would tell them he was starving and hadn't been given any food. His family complained, but no-one seemed to have the basic initiative to address a problem that could have been easily resolved. His relatives would go out and buy him food, or I would share the food my family had brought in.

The patients around me frequently soiled their bed because their requests for bed pans were ignored or action was delayed. These were elderly people who were unable to stand up for themselves. I witnessed nurses behaving aggressively and abusively towards these patients because of the mess they had created in soiling the bed. Several times, I intervened and tried to stand up for them.

These incidents greatly upset me, and I believe affected my recovery. I was becoming depressed from watching the appalling treatment of the people around me.

Late into one of the nights during my stay, the man in the bed beside me began falling out of bed. Because of his particular condition he was powerless to stop himself from falling. One of his legs had dropped out from under the bed covers and its weight was dragging the rest of his body off the bed. Feeling himself being slowly dragged, he pushed the nurse call button for half an hour before yelling at the top of his lungs to get a nurse.

By now everyone in our room was awake, and we all started yelling and pushing our nurse call buttons as we could see his dilemma. No nurses came, so eventually I had to lift myself into the wheelchair beside my bed, wheel myself to him, drag the table and chair beside his bed out of the way and hoist him back into bed.

After he settled down, I wheeled myself to the nurses' station. The response from the two staff on duty, who were sitting together not obviously busy doing something else, was that they had other things to do and would get there when they were ready.

I was continuing to suffer severe pain, and as changes were made to my medication, I became more aware that the source of the pain was my back. I was unable to sleep for more than a few hours at a time and could never get comfortable. I asked for, and received, an air mattress to help ease the pain but it didn't make any difference. My family brought in a soft mattress from home, which helped a little, but there was still no assessment and diagnosis of my spinal injuries.

Knowing now that my back was so damaged, it's clear I was more physically active in hospital than I should have been. I was using my upper body to heave myself from the bed to the wheelchair to get to the bathroom. Physiotherapists told me that to be discharged, I had to be able to get in and out of the wheelchair on my own and at least stay upright in the chair so

I could get from place to place. I was deliberately wheeling myself up and down the hallway for exercise, using the bed frame to do pull-ups to build up my strength and showering unassisted after staff set up a chair in the shower. These movements were further aggravating my back.

One physiotherapist, who appeared not to have read my chart, told me to try using crutches. Despite my injuries I was relatively fit and on heavy pain-killers, so I gave it a go. My legs swelled like balloons, and a surgeon came and told me my legs were not stable enough and using the crutches had caused internal bleeding.

Other doctors kept encouraging me to walk but didn't take into account that both knees were damaged. It was, "You've got a rod in there now, walk!" like the bone was as good as gold. Much later, at my own initiative, I saw a knee surgeon who told me my knee sockets were completely loose and my left hip had been pulled back out of its socket. In the hospital, no-one seemed to be seeing the whole picture.

During physio sessions they would try to get me walking using a frame. They'd help me to a wobbling standing position, then move the frame forward to encourage me to take two small steps. It was virtually impossible. Walking as I knew it was no longer an option.

I persevered because, more than anything, I wanted to get out of there and go home. I was frustrated that no-one would listen to me. Being on huge dosages of medication and getting contradictory advice at every turn was confusing and very stressful. I knew there was more wrong with me than the doctors and everyone else were conveying.

I came to realise one thing: it was up to me to take control of my recovery. As far as the health system was concerned, I couldn't rely on anyone else.

# Homecoming

**Mike**

Almost out of nowhere, hospital staff said to me, "Righto Mike, you've got two broken legs, we've put steel rods in them. Go home and your broken legs will heal up and you'll be fine, you'll move on with your life."

But moving wasn't really an option. I was in a wheelchair.

My homecoming was a blunt contrast to how I'd left only a matter of weeks earlier. Back then I was someone who was very fit and strong, at the top of my game in business and sport.

Suddenly, life was very different.

I lived in a large two-storey house with only narrow stairs connecting the ground level with the upper floor and the basement below. Luckily, the main bedroom was on the ground floor, which made access easier.

My family had a ramp installed so I was able to wheel my way from the driveway around the side of the house to the laundry door. It was a long route but I got used to it quickly and managed to get up a good speed.

I was incredibly fortunate that I had the use of my arms and could, after a bit of practice and with some help, manoeuvre myself from the wheelchair into bed.

The ground floor bathroom had a shower set into the bath, so modifying it with a seat was relatively easy. That allowed me to sit and have a shower on my own—luxury!

I'm pretty sure my kids made the most of the fact that I had no way of getting to their bedrooms upstairs. I've no doubt all manner of mischief went on up there while I was stuck down below.

While the experience of coming home in a broken state might have been overwhelming, I was still on strong medication, and a lot of my feelings were just not available to me. My care factor had diminished to virtually zero.

I was in this weirdly accepting state. I couldn't walk but I was so medicated I didn't understand how badly damaged I was. Actually, I didn't fully comprehend this for a long time. When I was discharged, everyone was still focusing solely on my two broken legs. I'd been monitored for a head injury, but there had been no specific diagnosis or treatment and it wasn't until much later that I discovered I'd broken my back in multiple places.

In between the drug doses, I was still in a huge amount of pain in my knees, hips and legs in general—and in my back, which at that time was still a mystery.

Neryl, my mother and other family members were so supportive I barely had to ask for anything. There were times I felt uncomfortable continually being waited on, but everyone was so accommodating it made it OK.

If I was stuck in the house for any stretch of time, I always had company. There were frequent trips to doctors and physiotherapy appointments, so we'd begin the ritual of leaving the house early to make sure we got there on time. Again, I was fortunate I had a Tarago van and the wheelchair could be folded up. I'd wheel my way around the house and to the driveway, then Neryl or Mum would help me into the van and wrestle with the wheelchair until it folded properly. Then they'd heave it into the back of the van and drive me to wherever we needed to go. At the other end, we'd go through the whole procedure in reverse.

As soon as I came home from hospital, my Dad arrived and said, "Mike, you've broken yourself. How are you going to get better? You're going to get better through exercise!"

Next thing, he'd built me a gym on the back deck of the house.

I had chin-up bars, weights and pullies—there were all sorts of exercises I could do from my wheelchair. I'd spend ages out there each day doing curls, press-ups, chin-ups and anything I could come up with to help make me stronger and accelerate my recovery.

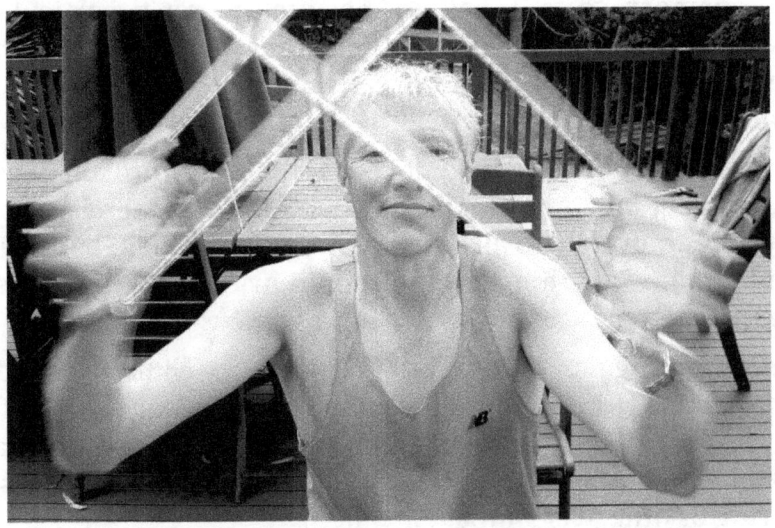

*Trying to build up my strength in my new outdoor gym*

Multiple blood clots had been discovered in my legs, so a nurse would come to my house twice a day to give me an injection of blood thinners to reduce the clotting. After a week I was told I'd have to learn to do the injections myself as the nurses weren't able to continue such regular visits.

I hated this particular routine. The needle had to be inserted into my stomach with a jab; it literally went in with a bang, followed by a painful press to get all the liquid in. I'd go to jab it in and my arm would automatically stop, because I knew it was going to hurt. Sometimes I had ten attempts before I could bring myself to do it.

Once I got the needle in, there was the awful sensation of the thick, cold liquid pumping in.

Every time I completed this process, it caused a bruise. After a while, the entire area across my stomach, from one hip to the other, was a series of bruises. It looked like I'd been kicked by a horse every day for weeks!

As a bonus, I also got to wear thigh-high white compression stockings on both legs to stop thrombosis. I was a picture of style.

The memory tests I had in hospital weren't particularly effective, given that the occupational therapists kept giving me the answers. It turned out I had swelling on the brain and my amnesia was severe.

I was more concerned about this than the broken legs. I knew eventually my legs would heal; I could exercise, go to physiotherapy and do all sorts of things to get them better. But I didn't know anything about brain injuries and how to make them heal.

I became a regular visitor at the brain injury clinic attached to Port Kembla Hospital, and this would continue for the next five years. They did a lot more testing to make sure I didn't have any ongoing brain damage that would affect my work skills or driving or otherwise impact my life.

While my memory now functions normally, I've never recovered my memories from the week leading up to the crash, the day itself and the weeks immediately after it.

Apart from my numerous medical appointments, I was something of a hermit during this period. Going out and socialising wasn't an option, but I had regular visits from my bike club friends. Sometimes they would call in as a group as part of a ride down the coast. At other times they would arrive in twos and threes or visit with their families.

## 5 | Homecoming

From being so much a part of the group, I was suddenly on the outside. They never made me feel that way, but the fact remained that I was a long way from being able to get back on a bike.

As the weeks of my convalescing stretched into months, I felt it was time for a foray into the outside world. Neryl and I were members of a business networking group that had black-tie meetings in the ballroom of a big hotel. We decided to try to get along to one of these meetings.

I struggled into a dinner suit and we did the whole Tarago routine so Mum could drive us to the dinner venue.

I remember wheeling myself into the pre-dinner drinks area where there was a big crowd, everyone done up to the nines. We'd both been out of circulation for so long it felt very strange to be there, particularly seeing it all from a seated position.

It was also an exhausting experience; in no time at all we were back on the phone to Mum and she was there to pick us up and take me back to bed.

### Neryl

It's hard to describe how different life suddenly became—thrust into running a busy household and being Mike's carer.

Mike and I had still only been together for a relatively short time. I'd got to know him as an extremely determined, confident and capable person; very fit, mentally sharp and full of every element of life.

Now he was physically broken, socially withdrawn as a result of the medication, clearly in constant pain.

Until that time, I'd never really considered the challenges faced by carers. I suddenly acquired an enormous appreciation for those who devote their time to caring for members of their family who are incapacitated in some way. I hadn't realised what an all-encompassing experience it was.

It's hard to imagine what it must be like for someone caring for a loved one in a wheelchair when there is no hope of recovery. And the challenges faced by older, more frail carers must be incredible. Even though I'm fit and strong, I often struggled to collapse or unfold the wheelchair and lift it in and out of the car. I certainly appreciated the disabled parking sticker that allowed us to park close to the door of shopping centres and other facilities. It was the only bonus, if you could call it that.

Grappling with the wheelchair and helping Mike in and out of the van when we were out in public proved to be an interesting social experiment. Lots of people were very caring and helpful; I had many offers of assistance and I started to notice a pattern in the type of people who would stop to help. Generally, people who were well-dressed or looked like they were on their way to work walked straight past us without making eye contact. More often, it was the individuals who were loitering about, more roughly dressed—those I would have probably tried to avoid talking to in other circumstances—who would ask if we were OK, if I needed help with the wheelchair or with Mike, and in some cases they'd get right to it and just take over the lifting process.

That was such a strong lesson for me; you can't judge a person's character by the way they look. The most unlikely looking helpers proved to be the biggest support.

It's staggering to think there are so many carers out there. In Australia alone there are more than 2.7 million unpaid carers, which is phenomenal. It's also a sad fact that many carers become ill because they don't look after themselves or don't have the opportunity to take regular breaks. We need to care more for the carers in our community.

Mike needed me and I was happy to be there. Things got a little more interesting when it came to being an instant stepmother to three young teenagers who lived with us every second week. It must have been so hard for them, seeing their Dad badly injured and now having to deal with me in the house. It was a big adjustment all round.

## 5 | Homecoming

Overnight, I went into a whirlwind of super-sized grocery shopping, continuous washing cycles, ironing school shirts and tunics (those darned box pleats!), cooking mountains of spag bol, shepherd's pie and all the other family staples, making lunches and ferrying very active teenagers to and from their busy schedule of activities—everything from scouts and circus training to drama classes and netball. Some nights I needed to be in three places at once and always managed to leave someone behind. We all did our best.

In between, Mike had plenty of medical appointments to keep us both hopping.

Taking it one day at a time is a well-worn cliché, but that's what we did. The one thing that kept me going was that I knew how determined Mike could be. Despite what some people were telling us, I didn't believe he was going to be in that wheelchair for long.

I've always had a healthy sense of humour, and while things seemed grim at times, there was always something to laugh about as well.

One source of amusement was the wee bottle—one of those hospital-issued plastic bottles that had, for some reason, arrived home with us among Mike's medication and hospital paraphernalia.

All the medication Mike was taking meant he had to be constantly hydrated, but manoeuvring out of bed in the middle of the night wasn't really an option, so the wee bottle became a permanent fixture.

Emptying it the morning was just one of the things I did—or sometimes Mike's Mum did—and it was task I quickly got used to. We've since joked it was lucky I knew exactly what it was, or I might have mistaken it for the worst Gatorade I'd ever tasted.

Later on, when our washing machine was playing up and we had to add extra water to the dirty clothes before starting the wash cycle, we discovered the wee bottle was the perfect implement to use. One day our cleaner saw it in the laundry and I'm sure became really concerned about what we were putting in the wash with our clothes.

## Mike

As time stretched on, the pain in my back was still excruciating. I had complained about it in hospital, but all they seemed to see at the time was my two broken legs.

Remember, I was pushing myself around in a wheelchair, lifting myself in and out of bed and doing a whole lot of exercise from the wheelchair, including chin-ups. I couldn't work out why my back was getting worse, not better.

My Dad had begun giving me regular back massages to try to ease the pain. One day he was rubbing my spine and exclaimed, "Mike, there's something wrong here. I can feel the bones moving under my fingers. It shouldn't be like this!"

Dad insisted I get it checked out. On his advice, we got in the van and drove to a local medical centre, where they had an X-ray facility.

I must have made quite a picture. After getting unloaded from the Tarago, I wheeled myself up to the shocked-looking woman behind the medical centre's front counter and asked for my spine to be X-rayed. I'm sure she thought it was a sick joke.

Eventually, I was seen by a doctor and repeated my request. He laughed in disbelief, joking, "What are you talking about? You've just come out of hospital, you've been there for about a month, you're in a wheelchair and you want your back X-rayed now? Get out of here!"

I had to insist something was wrong and I wanted it investigated, however bizarre the story sounded. "Look, I don't think it's been checked, and I can feel it's not right," I argued. "Will you please just X-ray my back!"

It took a while, but eventually I convinced him to arrange the X-ray. I was able to have it done on the spot, and the film was available straight away.

## 5 | Homecoming

When he received the X-ray, I can remember the doctor holding it up to the screen and looking at it for a long time. He was visibly pale. There appeared to be fear on his face.

Slowly, he pointed to not one, not two, but five broken vertebrae—one of them with shattered bone sitting behind my lungs.

He croaked out a nervous laugh, which quickly turned into an anxious instruction.

"You have to leave here and go straight back to the hospital! We're going to tear up these X-rays; you were never here. I won't put this on your chart at this clinic, as this should have been picked up at the hospital, and will have to be dealt with quickly."

"Tell them you need the X-ray and get them to look after you."

He was clearly frightened to have come across such an injury under those circumstances.

No wonder I was in so much pain! Dad took me straight back to the hospital, and I was X-rayed again. Those X-rays proved the fractures were there.

I was then bounced from radiographer to doctor to therapist—no-one knew what to do with me. My case had become a hot potato. They weren't prepared to recommend any treatment. Their best recommendation was that I shouldn't do any more chin-ups or strenuous exercise and to be very careful when lifting myself in and out of the chair.

Neryl called the office of the surgeon who had originally treated me, but the receptionist didn't want to give us an appointment. When Neryl used the words "missed injury", it was amazing how quickly an appointment became available.

I was referred back to the neurosurgeon whose clinician had assessed me in hospital and he advised that, considering I'd survived the accident and was already in a wheelchair, there was no specific treatment for the spinal injuries. Fat lot of help that was.

*Disrupt Your Life*

When I went back a few weeks later for a follow-up visit, his first question was, "How have you gone in your back brace?" I was staggered. I had never been given a back brace! I hadn't been offered any treatment at all.

Who knows what difference that would have made—would I have healed straighter? I didn't know it then, but the accident left me 2.5 centimetres shorter because my spine was compressed.

Considering the extreme pain I was in, it would have been a whole lot better to know about these injuries from the start. If you arrive at a major trauma hospital with serious damage from an accident, it seems reasonable to expect they will check you over properly. It's incredible to think that, even with the severity of my leg injuries, they never considered I might have spinal damage. Even though I complained of serious back pain, I was discharged from hospital untreated. It's a reminder that if something doesn't feel right, you need to persevere and keep asking questions until you get the information you need.

I started to become even more aware of the pain in my knees, hips and other places. I took things into my own hands and had more checks done.

I discovered I had hyper-extended both knees, snapping them backwards. As a result, both knee joints were completely loose, and the pain this was causing was horrific. This was never specifically identified or treated in hospital; their full focus was on the broken femurs. I was very lucky I didn't snap any of the tendons in the process.

My hips had also been damaged. I had to change a lot of the exercise regime I was undertaking.

The doctors started to change their story. When I was initially discharged from hospital, their line had been, "You've got steel rods in both your legs, it's time to go home and get better." Now, three months down the track, they were saying things like, "Michael, you've snapped your knees backwards, you've damaged your hips, you'll probably never walk properly again, you have a brain injury and you're going to have to take it easy because you've broken your back in five places. That's going to change your life forever."

They were saying this was going to have a profound effect on me and I was going to have to adapt to living a different life.

The psychologists at the brain injury clinic were singing a similar tune. They were telling me, "Mike, you're going to have to learn to live with this new body that's not as capable as it used to be."

Neryl had similar reactions from well-meaning friends and acquaintances. A neighbour who was a nurse commented, "I wonder how Mike's going to go when he transitions from being an acute patient with immediate injuries to having a chronic condition where he'll need treatment for the rest of his life."

Another friend took her aside and remarked that someone with two broken legs would never be the same. They had known someone in the past who had similar injuries, and, in their words, they'd "had it" as far as any hope of living a full life was concerned.

It seemed the expectation of everyone around us was that I was basically *cactus*—a shot unit who'd never be how he once was.

But I didn't believe that for a second. Every time I went to see the psychologist at the clinic, he'd tell me the same thing. Every time, I left with the same resolve: *I'm going to get better.* I've got broken bones and broken bones will heal. I've got good circulation because I keep fit and healthy. I will get better. I WILL get better.

But to be honest, things just got worse for the next couple of years, particularly with my legs. My back did settle down to some extent over a period of time, but my legs became more and more painful.

The road to recovery was just beginning.

# The long road

**Mike**

We had lodged a formal complaint about my treatment at Wollongong Hospital and my observations about how other patients were treated in the beds around me. As I mentioned in Chapter 4, we received a dismissive response; staff were interviewed but it seemed no action would be taken.

I felt gutted by the fact that I had been sent home from hospital with undiagnosed injuries. I worried about how much this might have set back my recovery; the stress that caused wasn't helping my state of mind.

Given my experiences with the health system, I considered legal action. I spoke to two different solicitors and both advised I had a strong case, not just for my treatment in hospital but also how my various injuries had been treated (or in many cases, not treated at all).

I thought about pursuing it but it just seemed too overwhelming, particularly as I still had a lot of recovering to do. A key element for me was that if I did go down the legal road, I would have to stay in a damaged state. I could only imagine what that would entail; I had visions of private investigators hiding behind trees outside my house taking photos of me. To win any kind of legal case I would need to demonstrate I had ongoing disabilities as a result of my treatment. I would need to look and feel injured for a long time.

That went totally against my inner determination to overcome my injuries. I was becoming fully focused on finding the right treatment, whatever that might look like, to move past the excruciating pain I continued to experience.

I started going to more and more physiotherapists and chiropractors to get different opinions. They would give me new exercises to try and I did them diligently, but the pain got worse rather than better. Without realising it, each exercise was creating more internal injuries.

Sheer persistence led me to gradually work my way from the wheelchair onto crutches. You wouldn't call it walking—more like inching along at a snail's pace.

My days were filled with physiotherapy sessions and aqua physio in Port Kembla Hospital's hydrotherapy pool, where I tried to do leg movements in the water.

I felt like a spring chicken at the pool. I was by far the youngest person doing rehab in the water, doggedly working through my exercises among all the hip and knee replacement patients.

I spent so much time there I made friends with some of the senior regulars, and we'd even go for coffee after our sessions.

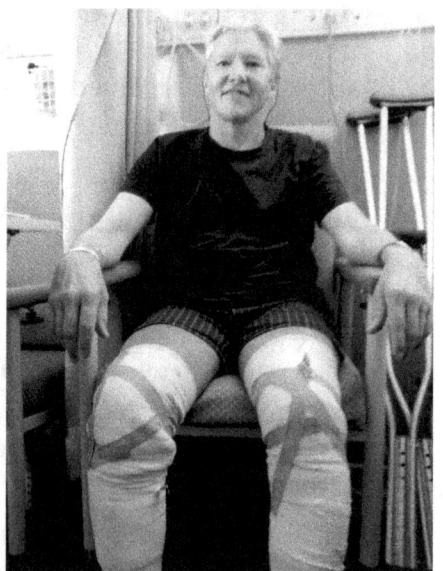

*Time to try to get mobile*

Eventually, I graduated from two crutches to two walking sticks—the type of canes normally reserved for old men. Neryl commented that me trying to walk with the sticks was like a drunken praying mantis, with more rocking than the Manly Ferry going through the heads.

## 6 | The long road

Life around me was slowly returning to "normal", whatever that meant for me now. I was still debilitated by pain, but I did my best to live with it.

On the toughest days—and there were quite a few of those—the one thing that really helped me was to focus on the people that needed me, rather than on my injuries.

I concentrated on being a dad my kids could be proud of. I wanted to show Neryl I was making an effort for her. I needed to keep my business running to maintain a roof over our heads—even though I was injured I still needed to pay the mortgage. There was no insurance to take the load off that responsibility.

Putting my attention on others gave me motivation to work harder at my rehabilitation. It gave me hope, something to look forward to, rather than thinking about what I had lost and how it might affect my life.

As part of trying to resume activities under this new normal, we decided to take the kids on a trip to Central Australia. I didn't want them missing experiences just because I had gone and hurt myself. The world had changed for them. Their Dad was crippled, Neryl was living in the house, we needed to give them a treat.

We got out and explored the sights every day of the trip. Some days were more difficult than others for me, but I wasn't going to let my injuries stop the rest of the family from enjoying the adventure.

We did quite a few kilometres of walking at Uluru and Kings Canyon. I was able to slowly hobble on two walking sticks by this stage, and I got confused looks from tour guides and other visitors as I tried to join in on the walking trails. A couple of times a guide intervened and told me I couldn't do a particular walk and would have to sit and wait for everyone to return, which I absolutely hated.

At one stage I decided to make a point of posing on a steep stone stairway at Kings Canyon, as if I was trying to get to the top. It was a set-up for the camera (and to get a reaction from the tour guide, which it certainly did), but it was also me saying, "Hey, I'm not going to let anything stop me!"

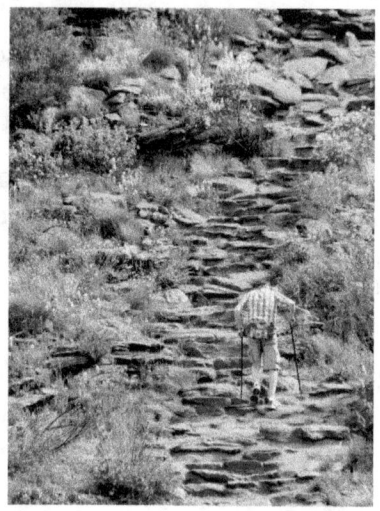 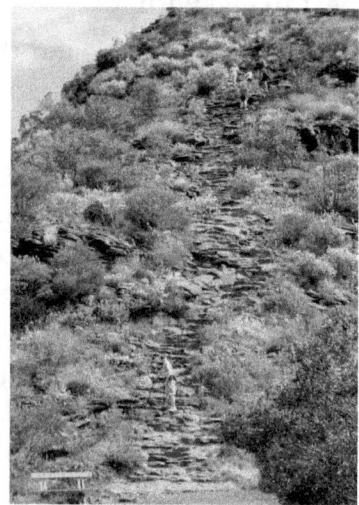

*I wasn't about to let anything stop me.*

Lots of things had to change for me. In my fibre optics business, I'd been the one doing the work on the tools. After the accident I could no longer do that—I wasn't able to stand for hours on end.

It had been a struggle to keep the business going, not only because of my physical injuries. The heavy pain medication meant I found it difficult to concentrate and make decisions.

I could have shut up shop, but instead I made the decision to take on staff for the first time. That was a whole new experience; until then, it had just been a part-time secretary and me.

Now I was employing more staff, I had to keep the projects coming in—which meant I had to somehow give potential customers confidence that my business could do the work. Sometimes that involved site inspections at coal mines or other heavy industrial locations. As the owner and technical expert, I had no option but to be the one doing the visit.

Rather than letting on how injured I was (and how much pain I was in, hobbling around on the site), I had to say I was disabled just so they would let me in the gate.

# 6 | The long road

On more than one occasion, I had to grit my teeth and cope with extreme pain while not letting my customer know how badly damaged I was. I couldn't afford it to affect my business.

The worst incident was a cave-in at a mine site, where I had to perform some emergency fibre optic repairs. I took an employee with me to help, but clambering over the rubble from the cave-in to fix the damaged equipment was extremely difficult. The pain was off the chart. I couldn't do anything for the next week while I recovered from that experience.

Another memorable day involved a site inspection in one of the busy railway tunnels under Sydney's central business district.

We accessed the railway line at the end of Town Hall station as soon as a train pulled out of the platform. That gave us one minute of inspection time before the next train came. We had to run along the railway line to a small alcove, wait for the train to pass, then continue on.

I was escorted by railway personnel so I had to look like I was fit for the task and pretended I didn't need sticks—but I was dying inside as I forced myself to shuffle along the track.

Despite those difficulties, the growth of the business opened up a whole new world. We took on some amazing projects, like connecting the fibre optics for the New Year's Eve fireworks on the Sydney Harbour Bridge.

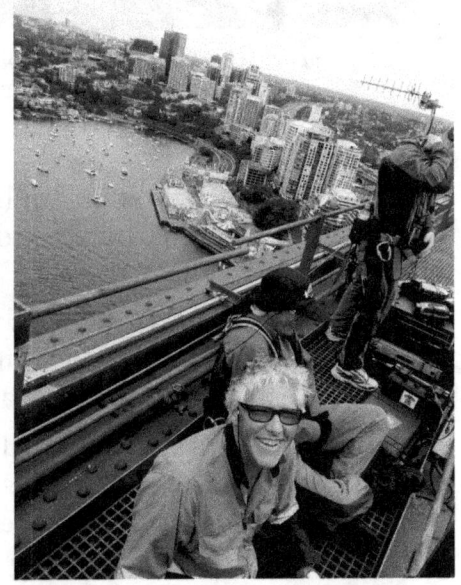

*Working at the top of the Sydney Harbour Bridge: the best view in town*

We also won national, state and local awards for our work, including Business of the Year in our region. I don't know if that would have happened if I wasn't faced with the choice of drastically changing direction with my business.

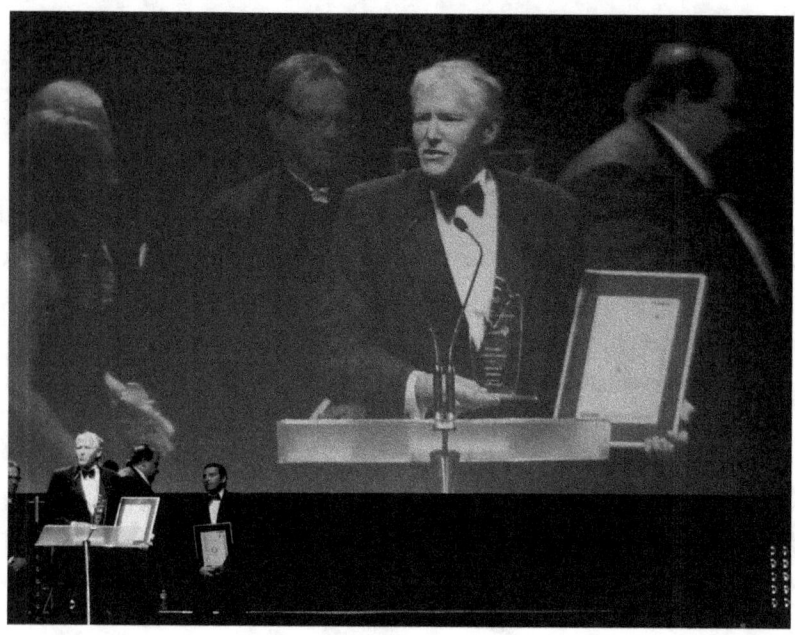

*The accident forced me to change my business approach and we went on to win multiple awards.*

## Neryl

A lot of people were telling us life, as we had known it, was over as Mike wouldn't be able to do the things he previously did. Mike didn't believe them.

Even though he kept a lot of this to himself at the time, he had a quiet determination about him. All the treatments, all the walking aides, were only temporary as far as he was concerned.

I'm sure they would have been telling anyone in Mike's situation the same thing, and I'm equally sure many people would have taken the advice as gospel and resigned themselves to a life of disability.

6 | *The long road*

There's a powerful lesson there; we must all be careful about what we say to people and, even more importantly, we need to take great care when it comes to the beliefs we take on from others.

In Mike's case, many of these opinions were coming from highly educated doctors. Some information conflicted with what he knew to be true. Even when advice comes from qualified people who are making their best judgement under the circumstances, we still have a choice about what we take to heart. You don't have to take the first opinion and run with it.

I'm not suggesting you disregard medical advice; there are many excellent medical professionals and we all rely on their expertise when we're sick or injured. But when it comes to big picture statements about your future and your life, you don't have to let negative predictions define what you do. It's about your own truth: what you know, deep down, you're capable of achieving, regardless of the circumstances.

I made a similar comment when speaking at a conference recently, and a surgeon in the audience pulled me aside afterwards. She challenged what I'd said, explaining that she and many of her surgical colleagues had been trained to paint a realistic picture for their patients, rather than raising false hopes. I told her more about Mike's story and she conceded that, in some cases, it would be better to empower patients with hope so they could make a choice about their own recovery.

In any event, it didn't matter what doctors and specialists told us—Mike was determined to recover and never once believed he'd spend the rest of his life with a disability. He made a different choice.

## Mike

The time since the accident was turning from months to a year. The pain in my back had gradually begun to subside, but both legs were still incredibly painful. I continued to take very heavy doses of morphine-based medication, which meant I was "off the planet" a lot of the time.

I had a weekend away with Neryl and I vividly remember being in severe pain the whole time. Trying to hobble down Pitt Street in Sydney, I more or less collapsed in agony. It was devastating—I think that's when it finally hit me that there was a lot more wrong with me than I was being treated for. I knew something had to be done.

By now, I was getting flak from some sections of the medical profession because of the number of avenues I was exploring to find out what was really going on with my legs.

One particularly narky physio threw at me, "You're just doctor shopping; you're not accepting anybody's advice." Actually, I agreed with her. I replied, "Yes, I am doctor shopping! I'm going to see as many people as I need to see, to get the answers that will get me better."

"Listening to you telling me I'm not going to get better, that I have to put up with this pain, isn't going to get me anywhere. It's not going to see me out for the rest of my life. So, if I need to continue to see doctors, I will see doctors."

Ultimately, my persistence paid off and some of the best advice came from the most unlikely people.

As a teenage apprentice, I had boarded with a Wollongong family. I hadn't seen their son for years, but he'd gone on to become an orthopaedic intern at Wollongong Hospital. I happened to run into him 12 months after the accident.

I told him about the intense, ongoing pain in both my legs and he had a look at my X-rays and other documents. His opinion was that the surgery on my left leg needed to be redone.

When the rod had been inserted, a six-millimetre gap had been left between the bones, which meant all my body weight was on the screws at either end of the rod. Over time, the screw holes had become elongated and the screws began to flex. That meant every time I took a step, the leg was contracting and expanding by up to six millimetres—a bit like walking on a pogo stick (if you don't know what a pogo stick is, you might need to consult *Wikipedia*). With this structure in place, my every movement was causing terrible pain.

In his opinion, the steel rod had to be removed, the ends of the bones ground back to promote new growth and the rod re-inserted.

This seemed to make a lot of sense. I went back to the original surgeon and he agreed to do the operation. After it was done, I checked myself into a specialist rehabilitation hospital. It was time to ramp up the action.

During my three-week stay at the rehab hospital, I was on an absolute mission to get better. I remember swimming laps with flippers up and down the pool and doing tricep dips and chin-ups. I was surrounded by elderly people and I was behaving like a full-on athlete. I must have seemed a total misfit. The physiotherapists became alarmed and told me to stop when they saw me "running" on a treadmill using my arms as support.

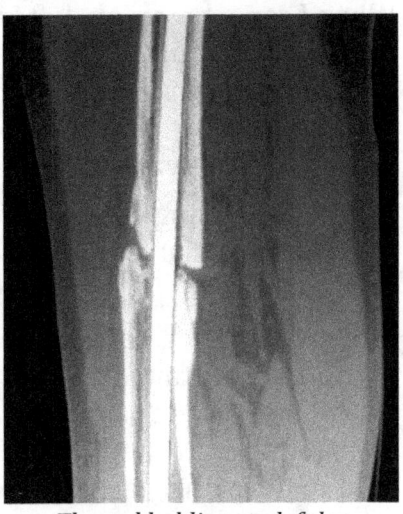

*The rod holding my left leg together*

Despite those exertions I made good progress with the rehabilitation of my left leg, but the pain in my right leg was becoming more acute. I had acupuncture in my right hip every day along with massages and cortisone injections, but nothing seemed to help.

This was another interesting reminder about our health system and how it can be difficult to have health issues treated holistically. It seemed I was only ever being treated for one thing at a time, even though I had multiple injuries. Staff at the rehabilitation hospital were well-meaning and gave me some treatment for my right leg, but they weren't particularly interested in finding the cause of the pain. They knew I was there because I'd just had new surgery on my left leg. Once they were satisfied with the left leg, I was discharged.

When I came home, my left leg was more comfortable as I was no longer walking on the "pogo stick" with my bones bouncing together. The engineer's brain in me said there was something seriously wrong with the rod in my right leg, but I was still unable to get anyone to look at it seriously.

Time was passing. It was hard to believe three years had now elapsed since that fateful day in 2010 when life as I knew it was disrupted.

I was continuing to explore every avenue of physiotherapy and other treatments to ease the pain in my right leg. One experience proved to be the straw that broke the camel's back. I'd been given a new set of exercises that caused so much additional pain even the morphine couldn't cover it. I felt absolutely desperate.

I dragged myself along to yet another doctor's appointment. I had to find someone who would take on my case holistically so all my treatments could work together.

The doctor wasn't quite ready to see me, but there was a young intern in his surgery who had a look at me while I waited.

He prodded and poked and asked me questions for about half an hour before the doctor came in. Then he said to the doctor, "Look, I think this guy's different. He's an athlete and I don't think we're in a position here to treat an athlete. I think we should send him to the Institute of Sport at Homebush. That way, he can be seen by someone who knows sports injuries better than we do."

That young intern was the first person who seemed to fully listen. He paid attention because, as it turned out, he had spent ten years as a personal trainer before going to medical school. He saw me as an athlete rather than a permanently damaged person. He could see past the injuries to who I was and respected that I did understand my own injuries.

Ironically, he was the least experienced of all the medical professionals I had seen. When Neryl and I speak about my story at conferences, we like to remind the audience that

## 6 | The long road

sometimes the best advice or inspiration comes from the most unlikely source. In your business or life, there might be people around you who have great insights and can solve problems, but they're overlooked because they're not considered to have the right qualifications or experience.

You never know, they might be the ones who have that one piece of information that's going to make all the difference. That was certainly the case for me.

The doctor took the intern's suggestion on board and referred me to a specialist at the Institute of Sport. Off I went to the Institute, where the specialist spent a long time examining me.

He was about to give his diagnosis without checking my X-rays, but I politely insisted he look at my latest films. I just knew something wasn't right.

He glanced at the X-ray of my right hip, rolled his eyes in shock and said, "I can't even diagnose you while this rod is in place."

The X-ray showed the rod in my right leg was sticking out the top of my femur by 40 millimetres. Every movement of my leg caught on muscles, tendons and nerves, which explained the agony I was in.

The exercises I'd been given were causing the steel rod to gouge into my hip bone from the inside.

The specialist gave me a referral to have surgery that would remove the rod from my right leg. His parting remark was, "If you think it's needed, come back and see me in two months—but with this removed I don't think you'll need to see me again!"

He was right. Within a week, I had the operation to take out the rod and the world was immediately a different place.

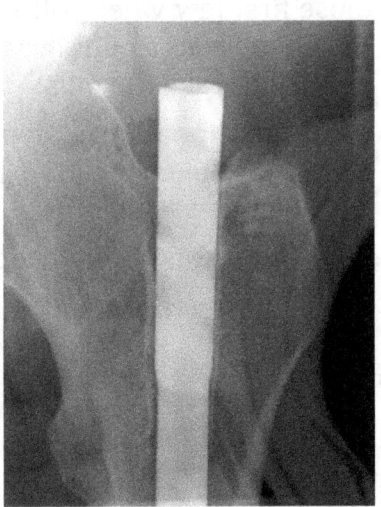

*The rod sticking out of the top of my right femur*

My life changed. My whole family's lives changed. Everything about what we were doing changed because the pain was virtually gone. All those years after the accident, it turned out to be the aftermath of the surgery causing the pain, not the broken bones themselves.

The words of the various specialists, psychologists and therapists rang in my ears. "You won't be able to walk properly again, it's unlikely you'll ever be able to run. Your physical strength and agility will never be the same."

I didn't believe any of them. I kept looking until I found someone who would listen to me. It took three years, but I found them.

The next decision I made was to go off the morphine-based medication. After the surgery to remove the rod in my right leg, I didn't feel the need for it any more.

I had been on very heavy doses for three years, but I stopped overnight. Specialists in the field will say you can't do that, you have to wean yourself off. I'm not recommending everyone goes cold turkey, but in my case I just made the choice and did it.

Neryl tells me there was a downside; I was pretty cranky in those first few weeks off the medication. She jokes that there were many occasions when she was telling me to "take the pills, Mike, take the pills!"

That lasted for about a month. I had some highs and lows while I came off the medication, but at last my mind was starting to feel like mine again.

The old me was coming back!

# The next three seconds—insights from Allan Parker

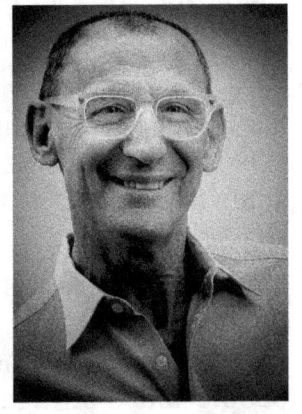

What are the differences between an individual who overcomes major injuries or other severe setbacks and a person whose life is derailed by negative circumstances?

**Micro-behavioural scientist Allan Parker** says the answer lies in a narrow window of time.

"Often people talk about *resilience*, yet I prefer the term *bounce back*, partly because I think resilience implies strength," he says.

"When we bounce back, we are not necessarily strong. The reality is we may even be desperately sore or weak or out of sorts; and yet when we get clear about making a decision to get up, and we do act on the decision immediately and move, irrespective of our undesired state, the bounce back is now real."

### Three critical seconds

"My research is about the choices we make **in the next three seconds**. Not, for example, 'Am I going to get up and go for a run?', instead 'I am going to get up now' and I get up now. And once I'm up, I take the next step and put on my running shoes and my shorts. And then I say, 'Now I am going for a run' and I do. It's clear, concise decisions about small things, decided and done frequently."

Allan says most people don't bounce back because, rather than making decisions about their actions in the next three seconds, they do it *across time*—projecting their mind from now to next week or beyond.

In the case of illness or injury that might involve them thinking, "I've got to get this sorted, I have to get back to work", but there are too many hurdles between their circumstances right now and work.

"For example, if I said to you, 'Let's go for a ten kilometre run,' there could be a very substantial part of you that responds, 'No, I can't do that, it's too much!'" he says.

"You can't even imagine yourself doing it, and by applying pressure I'm diminishing the chances of you succeeding. Whereas if I said, 'Let's go for a walk around the block and get some fresh air,' that's much easier for you to agree to."

"I've just asked you to go for a walk and you've said yes, so we have an agreement. But, we've still got to get shoes on and get out the door. There are still many decisions to be made. Rather than focusing on those three-second increments, too many people move straight to longer-term predictions, like where we're going and what the outcome is."

"The world is obsessed with goals, but instead it needs to be obsessed with *stages* and *behaviours*—and many decisions, not one." (For additional comments on the brain and goal-setting, read Dr Jenny Brockis' insights in Chapter 9).

Allan cites his experience of contracting a serious illness five years ago. As an ultra marathon runner, it took him two years to regain enough fitness to be able to run ten kilometres. His goal during that time was not to get *well*, but to *keep getting better*. The focus was on the moment-by-moment decisions that would keep him on track, not the end game.

# 7 | The next three seconds—insights from Allan Parker

For someone seriously injured like Mike whose story forms the core of this book—waking up in hospital and facing an uncertain future—Allan says there is little value in projecting beyond that crucial three seconds at a time.

"He can't improve if he doesn't stop and take stock of his body; how it feels and how it's functioning in that moment," he says. "If he rushes for improvement, he could put himself in danger. The wrong decision in those circumstances could take him backwards."

During a major life disruption, not everyone has the capacity to make helpful decisions in the next three seconds. If you're the carer, partner or friend of someone in that situation, Allan says the key is to give encouragement *in time,* not *across time.* Focus on the immediate choices in that moment, rather than longer-term "you can do it!" statements.

Practising small, positive choices in the moment builds lifelong habits that will come to the fore if you experience a major negative event in your life. "Knowing Mike's story, I imagine he had gone down into the pit and bounced back a substantial amount of times before his accident—which meant his brain and nervous system knew how to bounce back," says Allan.

Read more about the factors that help us bounce back in Sarah Boyd's insights in Chapter 11.

## Focusing out, not in

Allan says another major difference between people who bounce back and those who go backwards in time—affirming their pain, suffering and trauma—is that the ones who bounce back manage to get their attention *out of themselves* and into the external environment.

Focusing your attention inside yourself means you are fully present and involved with your current level of pain or discomfort. You're directly connected to your feelings and emotions. From this viewpoint, you see the world solely through your own eyes; this is where your sense of "self" resides.

Shifting your focus to how others see the situation, or how the situation might look to a third party, can give you a different perspective. Even in a three-second window, that can mean you make a different choice about what your next action will be.

"Let's imagine that, like Mike in this story, you're lying in bed badly injured," says Allan. "You're in a state of confusion because you have no clue about how you're going to progress or even if you're going to survive."

"All that intensity is going on, and then your partner arrives with loads of flowers and gifts for you. In that moment you have the choice of staying in your own experience or smiling and looking at the flowers and choosing to join your partner's experience."

"That's where the three seconds is critical. If you live outside three seconds, you can't have that level of awareness to make-well informed decisions about where you're putting your attention; inwards or outwards."

Most people go through life unaware that at any time they have the ability to consciously choose where their focus lies—and that a shift in perspective can make a profound difference.

## Your physical positioning matters

Allan points out that the human body has an in-built system to help us bounce back after physical injury, but sometimes we work against it.

"Dopamine and serotonin are neurotransmitters that make us feel good. Dopamine allows good thinking to take place in the frontal lobe in the brain," he says.

"Dopamine will transmit if the physical body is in balance. That involves the *vestibular system* — the sensory system responsible for providing our brain with information about motion, head position and spatial orientation that keeps you standing upright against gravity — and your *proprioceptive system*, which moves you and coordinates your muscles switching on or off so you can walk or run. If those systems are operating, your pain sensors won't be as active."

Having your feet on the ground or walking, slowly breathing in and out and having your visual attention outwards, will increase the likelihood of dopamine occurring — which means lying in a hospital bed is a biological disadvantage.

"That's why it's important to make sure a patient has a pillow or rolled towel under their knees so their knees are bent, taking the strain off their lower back, and that their feet are in touch with the bed surface, which will improve their breathing and increase dopamine," Allan says.

Allan put this into practice during the recovery from his illness. "You can't allow your body, emotions or mind chatter to determine how you're going to be. Most people think that's who they are—but that isn't the case."

"I would put my feet on the ground, take a breath in, breathe out and breathe in again, and on the third breath I made a conscious choice to feel composed. For 18 months I breathed in and out and chose composure at least 100 times a day."

"It wasn't to be composed for the next five minutes; it was to have the experience of composure *now*. Even if it only kicked in for two to three seconds, I acknowledged it and affirmed it. I kept reminding myself I would choose composure."

Managing three seconds at a time can keep you on the path of positive thought and action, even if the circumstances around you are anything but rosy. Small decisions, small steps acted on, produce bounce-back. This could be the pivotal factor in determining whether you stay stuck in a negative situation or choose to bounce back.

*Allan Parker mobilises human potential in individuals, teams and organisations by shifting the boundaries of possibility in thinking, strategising and behaving. More details at www.peakpd.com*

# New friends and giggly goals

**Neryl**

It had been remarkable watching Mike go from the wheelchair, to various forms of crutches, to two walking sticks, to one stick—and finally to a swaying shuffle all on his own.

He never said much about the extreme pain he was in throughout this time. He was dogged in his quest to get answers about why his legs didn't seem to be healing to a point where the pain was reducing. But otherwise, he did his best to pick up the life he had before the accident.

Of course, he couldn't do this completely. Getting around comfortably was an ongoing challenge and the medication interfered with his mental state.

Despite that, Mike's business continued to thrive, which absorbed plenty of our time. We also bought a house together in a dream location and began a major renovation (Mike jokes he agreed to the purchase while in a drug-induced state), so that also became a big focus.

That final operation, when the rod was removed from Mike's right leg, was the turning point. With the severe pain largely gone, along with the effects of the medication, he was able to get stronger. Little by little he began to lose the wobble in his walk. Today, looking at him, you'd never guess the extent of his injuries.

The day he took a few running steps was huge. We were on the beach near our house and I held Mike's hand as he completed a few tentative, wonky steps on the sand at a jogging pace. We chose a soft surface to avoid jarring.

He built up enough movement to let go of my hand and was able to run a few steps on his own. We both cheered!

We went to the beach a few days in a row, and he managed ten steps, then 20 steps and eventually he was able to run 100 metres. He was never going to be a threat to Usain Bolt, but it was a monumental achievement.

We'd managed to keep the business going and grow it considerably. Having no insurance claims or financial assistance was a big incentive to make it work.

In October 2013—just a few months after that final surgery—we stood on the stage at the Wollongong Entertainment Centre with our team as Mike's business was announced Business of the Year in our region. Looking out at that crowd of nearly 1,000 people as we accepted the award, I didn't imagine anyone in the auditorium had a clue about the struggle we'd been through to get there.

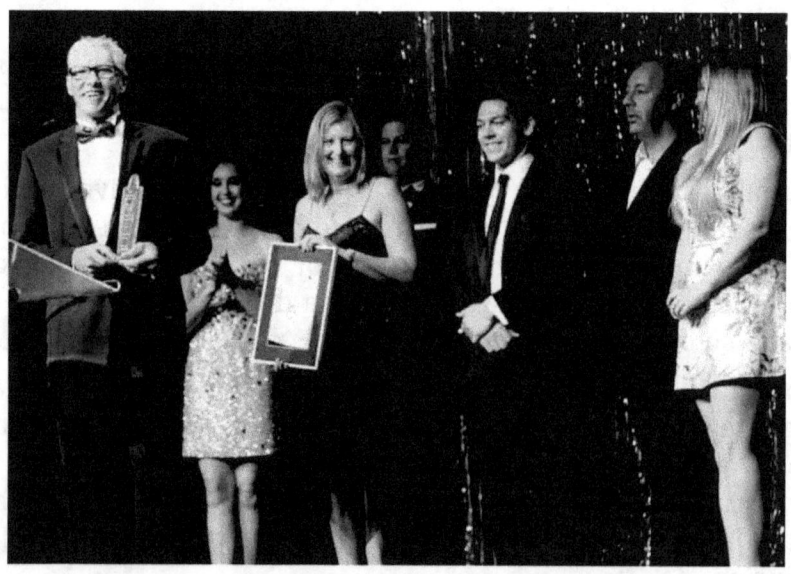

*Winning Business of the Year was an incredible moment.*

## 8 | New friends and giggly goals

After the years of turmoil since the accident, we were finally emerging on the other side. Our lives were different to how they'd been before that morning in 2010. In many ways—although we didn't fully realise this at the time—they were actually better. We'd moved to an amazing location by the beach, the business was going from strength to strength and Mike's physical state was improving by the day, now that the problem with the rods had been identified and addressed.

The one downside was he had lost the sport that had been his passion since childhood—motorbike riding. He still hung onto his bikes but they were gathering dust. I could understand why he didn't want to part with them, but he made it clear he had no intention of riding again.

That had a major impact on Mike's social life and his sense of belonging to a group, as most of his friends were in the bike club and based in Sydney. They remain friends to this day, but when the common thread between you is a shared activity and you can no longer participate, it's inevitable close friendships become more distant over time.

We sat down and had a specific discussion about this. Friendships had always been important to both of us, but with the frantic activity of our lives—between businesses and family commitments—we thought it might be difficult to create new friendships closer to home.

Mike was also looking for another sport; an outlet to replace the physical activity he'd enjoyed through the bike riding. Together, we made a decision about what would happen next.

Looking back, it would have been easy for Mike to sit at home and expect his bike club mates to take time out of their lives and travel to Wollongong to visit him, even though he no longer shared that common focus. He could have felt sorry for himself and focused on the things he could no longer do. Instead, we decided to do something different, and we acted on that choice.

The power of making clear choices and following through with action has made a massive difference to both our lives. You might catch yourself saying, "I'd like to do this," or "one day I will do that". Until you get clear and make a decision to start, those are only vague dreams.

> "The most difficult thing is the decision to act, the rest is merely tenacity." - Amelia Earhart, who in 1932 was the first woman to fly solo across the Atlantic.

## Mike

I'd been dabbling in the sport of surf ski paddling for a while before the accident. In fact, you might recall from Chapter 3, on the morning of the crash I had intended to go paddling and changed my mind at the last minute to go riding with my mates instead.

I loved being in and on the ocean. It was a fun way of keeping fit and there were some amazing people involved in the sport, with a shared passion for getting out on the water.

After the accident—and before the surgery that corrected my right leg—I had tried to paddle a ski again, with limited success. I was still in a lot of pain at the time and found it very difficult, not only when I was on the water but also trying to get out of the boat. Despite that, I pushed myself and had a go in a couple of smaller surf ski races on flat water.

After the rod was removed, I tried again and found that I was able to improve because the pain had eased considerably. I was still at a beginner level and wanted to take it up more seriously. After discussing it with Neryl, I decided to make this new sport a focus.

While the sport itself was important, a big factor in the decision was that taking up paddling seriously would involve a whole new circle of friends. The local Wollongong paddling group included some of the country's—and world's—best paddlers, as well as those at beginner level and social paddlers. The more serious paddlers trained hard most mornings of the week and

## 8 | New friends and giggly goals

there were also plenty of gentler paddles and informal get-togethers.

The group welcomed me from the start, even though I was probably the slowest paddler of all of them and fell out of the boat multiple times every training session.

My decision not to ride bikes any more was made out of respect for the people around me. If I'd wanted to, I could have worked my way up to sitting on a bike again.

I still had a BMW 1200 GS, which is a large off-road adventure bike, and a BMW 650 dirt bike which had been set up for competition and desert racing. They were slowly rusting in our garage, and my cupboards were still full of riding gear.

I had plenty of mates who would have gladly ridden with me. But I chose not to do it. Neryl had spent enough time pushing me in a wheelchair. My parents and kids had suffered enough through my recovery.

As part of my treatment, we also discovered I had low bone density as a result of coeliac disease. In fact, I had osteoporosis, which meant any fall from a bike would lead to injury. I realised it would be unfair on my bike club mates for me to ride with them. If I were to fall off the bike, even in a minor way, I would almost certainly break multiple bones.

In making this decision it wasn't like I sent my motorbike mates an email that said, "That's it, you're dead to me!" They are still my friends and always will be. But I wasn't one of them any more. I wasn't about to jump on a bike any time soon.

By committing to the paddling group, I made many new friendships. We'd go paddling together, then have a coffee or meal. When we went to races we'd organise buses and trailers and travel together. It opened up so many doors for me.

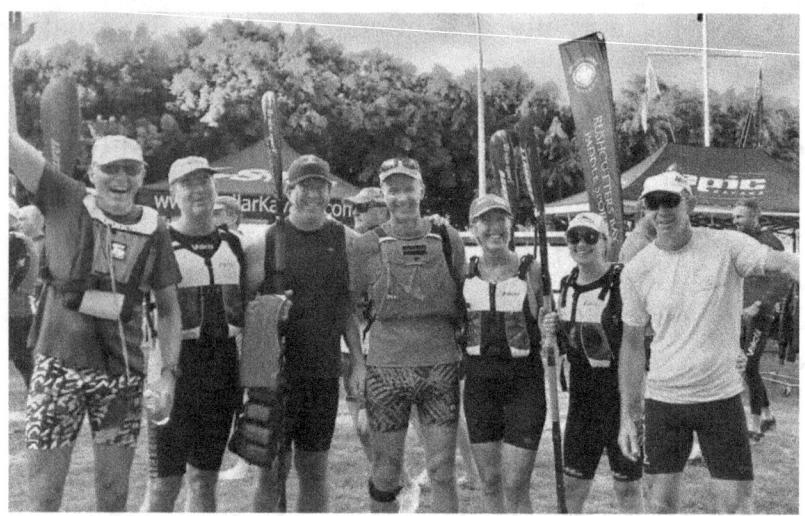

*I found a new circle of friends in the Wollongong Paddlers.*

Of course, I had to build up slowly. When I joined the group, they had some idea about my situation although they didn't realise the full extent of my injuries. I look back on some of those early sessions and cringe, because I was definitely not a good paddler. That didn't matter to them; they supported me right from the beginning.

There were times when I would be out on the ocean and, because of the back injury, one side of my body would seize up. I would be frozen and unable to move, which isn't a great state to be in when you're sitting on what feels like a round log on a bumpy ocean.

Someone from the group would always be by my side, making sure I was OK. Slowly, they'd help me back to the shelter of the harbour.

At other times I couldn't hold up my own body weight after paddling for an hour or so. I would have to deliberately fall out of the ski in deep water, float myself to the beach and slowly hobble up the shore, dragging my boat behind me. I must have been a pathetic sight. But the other paddlers were patient with me and gave me lots of encouragement.

## 8 | New friends and giggly goals

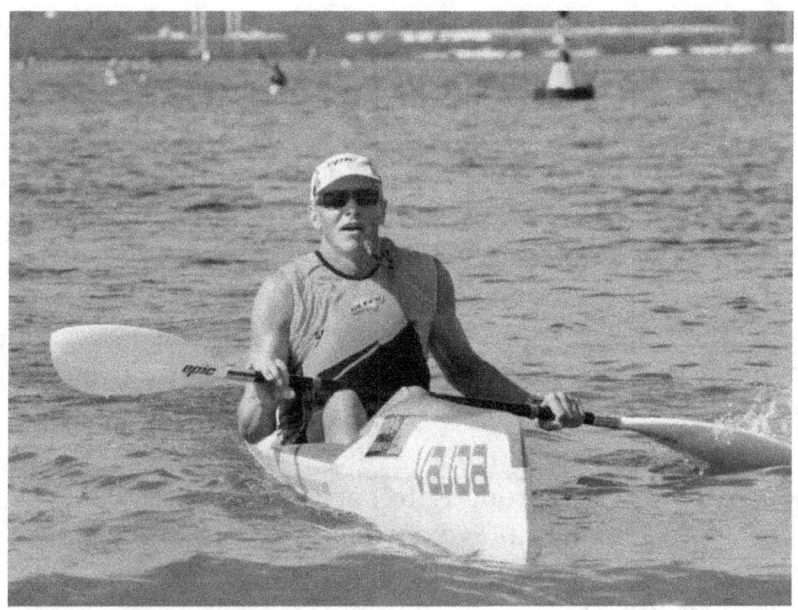

*One of my early paddling races: my face says it all*

I didn't see paddling as a weekend hobby. I wanted to learn to do it really well so I could become competitive in races. I hadn't realised it when I took up the sport, but ocean ski paddling has a worldwide following and a busy calendar of international competition.

It's a remarkably technical sport; my first big lesson was that, even though you're using the paddle to drive the ski through the water, it isn't an "arm" sport. The hand holds the paddle but all the strength comes from rotating the body through your core. This is a difficult concept to master.

As a child, I remember Mum telling me never to be afraid to ask for directions, and I put that philosophy to good use in increasing my paddling skills. I sought out some of the champions and legends of the sport, including former Olympic kayakers, and found they were incredibly generous with their time and knowledge.

I went to a training camp at Ningaloo in Western Australia and spent an entire week with Dean Gardiner—multiple world paddling champion—and other coaches who were ex-Olympians. I had intensive coaching from Oscar Chalupsky, a South African and giant of the sport who is a genius at reading ocean conditions. Neryl tells me I came back after that session with eyes as big as saucers, like I'd been infused with some energy drug. Whenever there was an opportunity to attend a coaching clinic I went along and soaked up all the expertise like a sponge.

It was more than a sport; I became part of the bigger paddling community. After a few years of paddling, I felt part of a global movement.

It was wonderful to become strong enough to compete properly in surf ski races, locally and in Sydney. Just being part of it was great, although I could feel the return of my old determination to do better and better.

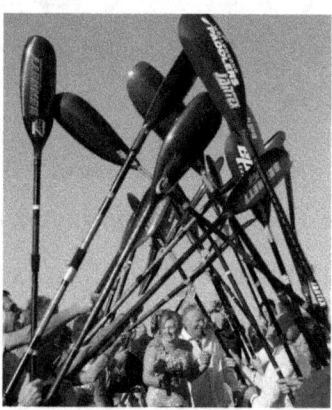

*Our paddling friends played an important role at our wedding in 2014.*

While most of the races had a finish line in the water, sometimes there would be a beach sprint at the end, and that posed a problem for me. I was now walking with relative ease, but I hadn't progressed to running competitively—especially on soft sand!

In those early events with a beach finish, I had no choice but to roll out of the boat at the end of the race, pick up my paddle and use it as a crutch as I hobbled up the sand to the finish line.

Sometimes the crowd would make a point of cheering me on—like that swimmer at the Olympics everyone feels sorry for and cheers for coming last.

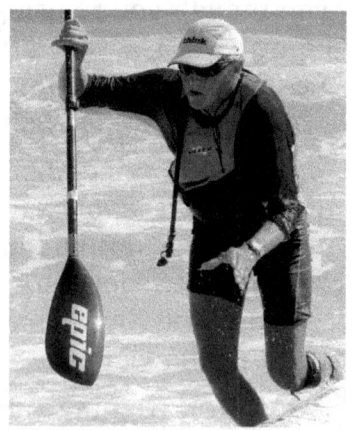

*My race finishes weren't a pretty sight.*

I'd be lying if I said there weren't times I wanted to give up. Finding the motivation to train for races when I was still feeling the effects of my injuries, unfit and overweight, was really difficult.

With the support of the paddling group and my family, I gradually reconnected with the inner drive that compelled me to keep going.

My paddling results steadily improved. I entered more races and stretched myself to finish in the top ten. I felt less like an injured person undergoing rehabilitation and more like an athlete training for bigger results.

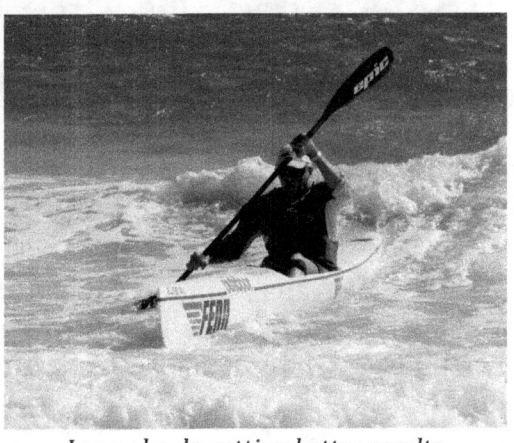

*I was slowly getting better results.*

By now I was in my fifties, and if you're thinking that seems relatively old for competitive sport, you'd be wrong when it comes to ocean paddling. The fifties age group is the biggest and most hotly contested category in paddling races around the world. The best male paddlers in their fifties, including Dean Gardiner and Oscar Chalupsky, consistently finish in the top ten of the open field, leaving most of the younger paddlers in their wake.

The international paddling calendar included races in some magical locations, like Mauritius, Hawaii, Canada and Portugal. While Neryl isn't a paddler, we joke that she's gone from supporting me and my bike riding by camping in dusty bush locations, to enjoying being part of the paddling community at some of the most spectacular places on earth.

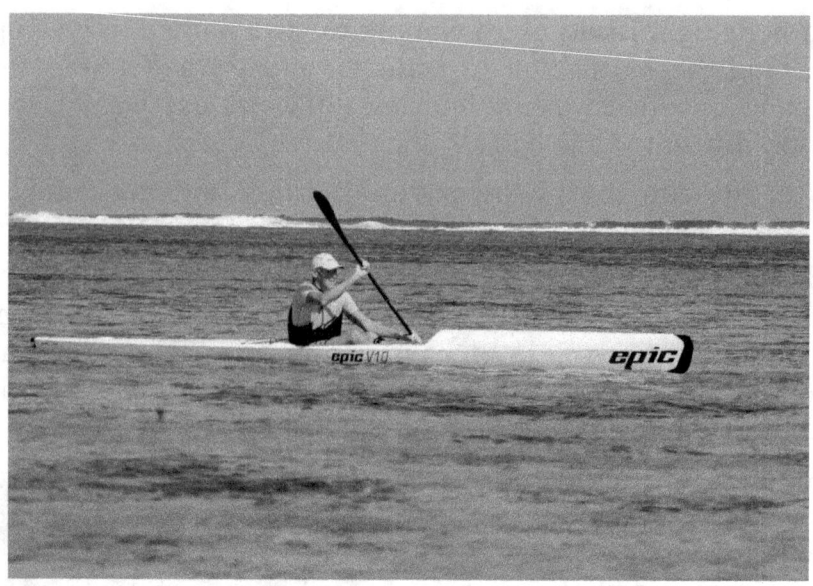

*Competing in spectacular Mauritius*

As I continued to get stronger, I decided to enter one of the world's most legendary races, The Doctor. Named after Western Australia's famous Fremantle Doctor afternoon wind, it's a 28-kilometre race from Rottnest Island, off the coast of Perth, to Sorrento Beach across waters famous for their shark infestation.

It was incredibly exciting to get a start in such a huge international race, and it also proved to be a massive learning curve. I fell out of the boat three times during the race, got lost and headed for the wrong beach.

Still, I persevered and finished the event. I was determined to race as much as I could until I could compete without falling in.

## 8 | New friends and giggly goals

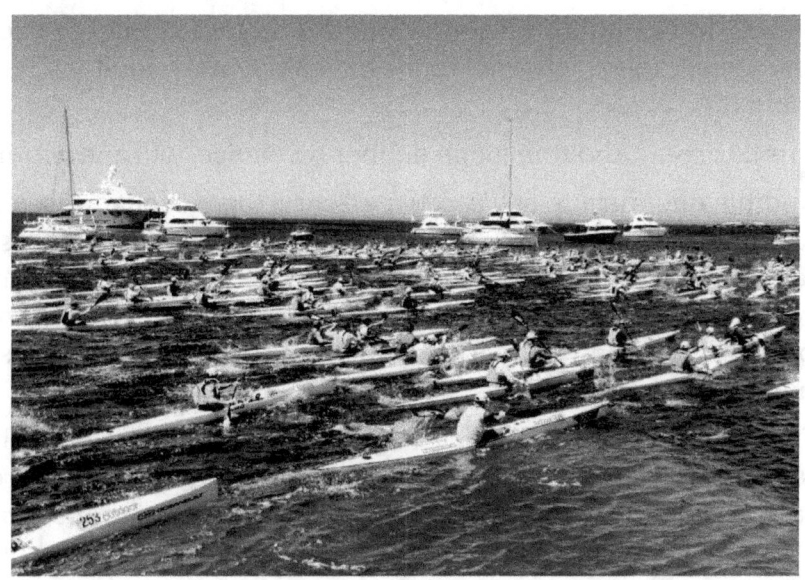

*The start of the legendary "Doctor" race*

As if The Doctor wasn't big enough, I took up an opportunity to compete in the Molokai Challenge, another legendary event involving a race across 53 kilometres of open ocean between the Hawaiian islands of Molokai and Oahu. I knew it was out of my league as a solo competitor so I did it as a relay, which enables you to race as a tag-team with another paddler. I thought this would be a great way of learning about the event, with a view to possibly doing it solo in the future.

As a relay team, we were each supposed to paddle ten kilometres at a time. The paddler not on the water travelled on an accompanying support boat until it was their turn to compete again. In our case, my paddling buddy broke a rib while getting into the support boat at the very start of the race and was only able to complete five kilometres on each of his stints. I ended up doing 40 of the 53 kilometres. So much for a learning experience!

Our lives could so easily have shrunk after the accident, but in fact our world has expanded. I've become more involved in the business community. We have an incredible circle of friends. My paddling has helped me get fit and strong. My back has healed amazingly well and I haven't overstrained my legs doing it.

This has come about through deliberate choice, will and action.

Finding out during my recovery that I had coeliac disease has potentially added 20 years to my life. This diagnosis also helped my paddling, because I was able to adjust to a gluten-free diet, which enabled me to absorb more energy from my food. Despite the very dark days I went through, there are so many positives.

If you're in a difficult place in your life right now, it might be hard to see the possibilities—but they're always there. Regardless of the circumstances, you have a choice about what you believe in your own mind. You can make a decision about how you will respond.

> "Everything can be taken from a man but one thing: the last of the human freedoms—to choose one's attitude in any given set of circumstances, to choose one's own way."
>
> "Between stimulus and response there is a space. In that space is our power to choose our response. In our response lies our growth and our freedom." – Viktor Frankl, psychiatrist and Holocaust survivor

## Neryl

It was now six years after the accident, and we made some new choices about the next phase of our lives.

I'd become fascinated with the psychology of goal-setting; what can be achieved when we get specific about what we want and take daily action towards it. As part of this voyage of discovery, I had become a coach in a program called YB12, which stands for Your Best Twelve Months.

## 8 | New friends and giggly goals

YB12 has an excellent suite of programs for groups and individuals, all around beating procrastination and managing the parts of your mind that hold you back from achieving results. They also have a specific process for setting your goals and breaking them down into bite-sized, achievable actions. You can see more about YB12 at www.yb12coach.com.

I was delivering a YB12 workshop called Total Focus, part of which involved participants setting out the results they wanted to achieve to enable them to have their best year. It was my first public outing with this program and I wanted good numbers in the room, so I asked Mike to join in.

When we got to the goal-setting part of the session, he came up with what I would call a *giggly goal*—one of those huge, sweeping statements you say you're going to go for, but you can't say it without laughing. It's just too big and scary.

He had mentioned this idea in passing before, but I had never taken it seriously. This was the first time he articulated it fully and thought about the actions required to achieve it.

This was the giggly goal: Mike wanted to make the Australian ocean racing team in the hotly contested fifties age group and compete at the world championships for ocean ski paddling.

The next world championships were to be held in Hong Kong in 2017. It was clear Mike *really* wanted to get on that team, but at the same time it seemed crazy.

The guy known for being in the wheelchair, having a broken back, hobbling up the beach using the paddle as a crutch—to be representing Australia in one of the most competitive categories of his chosen sport?

I didn't want to be negative about it, but at the time it didn't seem realistic.

Mike being Mike, he made it his mission anyway. It didn't matter to him if it seemed nuts. Giggly goal or not, he intended to go for it.

# Superpowers and a state of thriving—insights from Dr Jenny Brockis

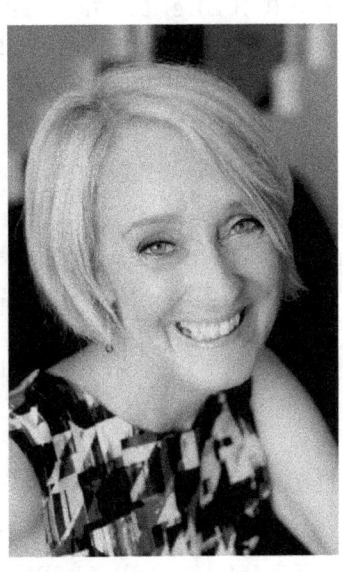

Are you thriving in your life or merely surviving?

Thriving has been described as reaching your highest potential, regardless of the circumstances around you. Surviving, on the other hand, is about staying alive or continuing to exist, especially under adverse or unusual circumstances.

Actively moving towards a state of thriving, where you're doing more than just continuing to live and breathe, enables you to manage life's disruptions more effectively. But how can you do that? And why does it seem to come more naturally to some than others?

**Dr Jenny Brockis** is a medical practitioner, award-winning speaker, trainer and facilitator who—through her business, *Brain Fit*—helps people understand why they think and act the way they do, and implements science-backed behaviour change to turn around some of the biggest performance issues in organisations.

She believes the frantic pace of life and our fixation with technology means we're depriving ourselves of opportunities to thrive, which can have serious consequences if we face a life disruption that's not of our choosing.

You might have an intention to feel good, enjoy what you're doing and focus on staying calm and contented, but that can be outweighed by a fear of not keeping up.

"We've got stuck on the survival treadmill and it feels too hard—and perhaps too dangerous—to step off and try a little more thriving," Jenny says. "We believe we have to keep our heads above water—we worry that if we stop pedalling, we'll drown."

While it might make our life easier in some respects, obsessive use of technology actually makes our brains work faster and has been shown to contribute to an increasing sense of "time poverty".

In such a busy world, an unexpected challenge can tip us over the edge.

"That's why some people end up just keeling over," Jenny says. "When you've got so much on your plate and you're trying to juggle everything at the same time, if something tragic happens it can feel as if you've got nothing left in your tank to deal with it."

## How to move towards a thriving state

One way to help yourself thrive is to **take "digital detox" breaks;** to step away, switch off the technology and allow everything to settle down. That process helps reconnect you to the idea that you do have enough time—it's how you choose to use it that counts.

**Regular meditation** helps you step off the treadmill, relax and breathe, producing a calming effect where stress levels fall.

"And all of a sudden, it's like it opens up this lovely new world and you think, 'Ooh, this feels good!'" says Jenny.

**Be aware of what you say to yourself** and how you talk about yourself to others; this can reveal the hidden beliefs that stop you thriving and drain your resilience tank. Not being aware of these limiting beliefs magnifies their power and allows you to hold on to them.

In Jenny's experience, people who thrive have limiting beliefs like everyone else. The difference is, they are aware of them and can address them in the moment rather than letting those beliefs cripple their actions.

"The common thread, where some people have broken loose, is simply developing that self-awareness," she says.

"These beliefs have usually evolved from childhood experiences—how we're brought up, how we were taught to behave in certain situations, what the response was if we did something wrong, how we were punished and so on. Our beliefs evolve and develop as we grow older, unless we challenge them and question their validity."

**Take small steps to shift your feelings**, especially when you know you're stopping yourself from achieving your goals—for example, sabotaging your efforts to go to the gym by coming up with excuses or sleeping in.

"You might think, 'I'm fed up, frustrated because I understand if I apply myself differently, I'll get a different result.' But how can you do that?" Jenny suggests you step back and ask, "What am I telling myself here? And if I don't like the way it's making me feel, what can I do differently?"

One small action can shift you towards a more positive outlook.

"This is the critical thinking phase, which in the modern world we often don't take time out to apply to ourselves. If you find yourself saying, 'I couldn't possibly do that' or 'I'm too old' or whatever, take the time to ask, 'Hang on a minute, where's the truth in that? Is it valid, is it relevant to me and how do I feel about that?'"

"If we don't tap into our feelings around these beliefs, we can't consciously mould them into more helpful thoughts that will bring a more positive outcome for us."

**Spend time with people who challenge your limiting beliefs.** Catching and questioning negative beliefs can be difficult on your own, and they can be contagious in the wrong company. It's important to hang out with people who don't share the same self-limiting beliefs as you. Talk to someone who will support you but also hold you accountable. If they hear you using self-defeating language they might say something like, "Stop talking like that! It's not true!"

**Stop telling yourself horror stories.** Often the stories we tell ourselves about an event (the "meaning we make from it", as Sarah Boyd phrased it, see Chapter 11) are far worse than the actual incident.

Even specialists in the field can fall for this one. Jenny describes how a friend she works with on a mentoring basis recently sent her a string of emails cancelling every catch-up and phone call they had scheduled for the rest of the year. "My response was, 'What have I done? I must have upset her in some way'," she says. "I spent five days thinking I was a terrible person. I fixated over what could make her behave like this, what I had done wrong."

"I tried to reach out and she didn't respond which, of course, fuelled my self-limiting belief that I had somehow offended her. It turned out there was a glitch in her email system, which led to the string of cancellations. She was totally unaware it had happened."

Rather than jumping to conclusions and having sleepless nights as a result, we can allow the logical part of our brain to challenge our assumptions—which in this example might lead us to investigate what's really going on.

"Even though I knew there must have been a logical explanation, my belief system was still set up to take over and create the drama and the story," Jenny laughs.

## 9 | Superpowers and a state of thriving—insights from Dr Jenny Brockis

"We're so good at creating these narratives for ourselves. If you recognise you're a bit of a catastrophiser, you can do a self-intervention and recognise those type of thoughts don't help anyone—and the person they help least is you."

### Using your superpower

As a medical professional working in the area of brain science, Jenny marvels at the ability of humans to *think about our thinking*; to apply conscious thought and choice to what we're doing.

As you will see from the story of *Disrupt Your Life*, the daily thoughts, seemingly insignificant choices and actions we apply make a huge difference to the direction of our lives.

At other times we can consciously choose to make larger changes that enable us to move towards bigger goals or away from situations, behaviours or people that are holding us back.

Jenny cites the case of a young man she met recently who had a very troubled past: subjected to abuse in a dysfunctional family, falling in with the wrong crowd and getting mixed up with drugs, fathering a child at a young age and ultimately ending up in jail.

In prison, he took stock of his life and reflected that, "so far, it's been pretty sucky". While many people in those circumstances are almost resigned to the fact they're going to continue on a similar path, this individual made a conscious decision it wasn't going to be like that for him.

He decided it was time to clean himself up, stay sober and change his relationships by ditching the unsupportive ones and finding new people to hang around with. While this wasn't easy, he achieved his goal by focusing on his newly found self-belief and keeping himself accountable.

"I really believe the ability to consciously choose is our superpower," says Jenny. "When you hear a story like that, it's the superpower of our conscious mind that enables us to step up."

"The beauty of this example is that not only did he have the insight that he could change himself, but he could also influence others who might be stuck in that same place. He helps them think through things in such a way that they feel enabled or empowered to make that choice for themselves."

## Balancing the roles of our brain

Your brain has a critical role in keeping you safe at all cost, which is why it can feel so challenging to move out of your comfort zone into something slightly risky. But there's also the other aspect of the brain; the part that wants you to feel rewarded.

Those two elements can sometimes feel at odds; you want to take on a new challenge or make a change, but your safety-conscious brain steers you back to the status quo.

Jenny says the key is getting the two to work together. This involves recognising the power of your feelings. Every thought is influenced by the emotion associated with it at a subconscious level. Recognising the emotion, and the feeling it gives you, can help shift your thinking. Focusing on positive emotions and feelings associated with what you want to achieve can, over time, override the brain's urge to keep you safely where you are.

"I talk about this with business people all the time because they're applying logic, analysis and reasoning to their decisions and often say there's no room for emotion in business," Jenny says. "I tell them, 'Well actually, every decision you think you make with your rational mind is actually underpinned by the feeling associated with it'."

So, is it possible to move beyond your current circumstances to achieve goals you've previously struggled to reach? Absolutely, if you're prepared to take on the challenge of rewiring your brain.

"Some people go through life obliviously and that's their choice—and you're never going to influence them to think differently," Jenny says. "On the other hand, you can choose to rewire your thinking. It will take effort, energy and time because it doesn't just happen overnight."

"You're literally changing your neurobiology, because changing your mind requires the creation of new connections between your brain cells, which through repetition and practice become strengthened and embedded as new neural pathways and your new default way of thinking."

We spend a lifetime evolving our pathways until they become superhighways running through our minds. It can take effort to build a new superhighway that will become the path of choice that the brain goes to in a particular situation, rather than defaulting to the old one.

"We talk about breaking habits, but we don't need to break them at all; we just have to stop using that particular way of thinking that's holding us back and replace it with a new way which can only get stronger by going back to it and practising it more and more," Jenny says.

While you might have seen ads that spruik slogans like *21 days to a new, beautiful you*, Jenny says the reality is it takes an average of 66 days—even up to a year—to develop a new way of thinking.

"We all have lapses and relapses when making conscious changes in our lives," she says. "Each time you practise and go to the new route, you'll get better at it. The old route never completely goes away and when you face adversity your brain goes straight back to the old way because it doesn't take as much energy as the new one."

"That's the third priority of the brain—to conserve energy, no matter what. So, if it has the easy option, it will always go there. That's why we fall back into old habits and assumptions and jump to conclusions. It doesn't take nearly as much energy to do that."

## Can everyone learn to disrupt their own life through conscious choices?

While there are those in the world who seem to automatically veer towards enjoying life and getting the most out of it with ease, they are, in fact, applying conscious effort.

"It's something we all have to deal with in our own way, and while some people may be perceived as having an easier route, I believe no matter who you are, everybody has to work at it," Jenny says.

She gives the example of a friend of hers who seems to have it all—great career, athletic ability, a giving nature, huge involvement in the community. It's easy to look at this person and think, "You are truly thriving. You are living the life that I aspire to."

"But, I know it hasn't just happened to her," Jenny says. "This is something she's evolved gradually over a period of time because it not only gives her pleasure, she also finds it rewarding."

"When we do something inherently rewarding, our brain responds with, 'Ooh, nice!' and releases dopamine."

Dopamine, which we mentioned in Chapter 7, is commonly associated with the brain's pleasure and reward system. Neurotransmitters are chemical messengers which facilitate communication between nerve cells in the nervous system.

"That dopamine hit, in turn, motivates us to repeat that behaviour. It then becomes self-perpetuating because the more we repeat that behaviour and get the outcomes we desire, the easier it is to keep moving forward on that trail."

"So, the key is, 'more dopamine, please'."

## The brain and goal-setting

When it comes to setting *giggly goals* like the one we refer to in Chapter 8, the brain can work against you unless you break the big goal down into small, manageable chunks.

## 9 | Superpowers and a state of thriving—insights from Dr Jenny Brockis

"Basically, humans are very short sighted," Jenny says. "We've evolved to think about what's happening right now and what might be happening in the next five minutes, the next day or the next couple of weeks."

"The longer-term view is something the brain doesn't feel comfortable with because it's abstract. The brain likes the concrete, the certainty of exactly what the future will look like—and we can't produce that because we don't know."

"When you think about yourself right now, you're using a certain part of your brain. If you think about someone else, you're using a different part of the brain. When you picture yourself in the future, it's as if you don't recognise yourself—you're seeing yourself as someone else—so you're using that different part of the brain. The brain really struggles because you're trying to think about yourself in the future but the picture doesn't match."

Setting goals becomes a whole lot easier when you know how to work with your brain to make it happen.

"A lot of people work in 90 day sessions for goals; it's about making it manageable so the brain can have the certainty it's looking for," Jenny explains. "The brain is a prediction machine; it likes to predict how things will turn out."

You can help activate your "prediction machine" by:

- Having a very specific goal.
- Writing your goal down—the act of writing helps to embed the goal in your brain.
- Breaking your bigger goal down into small pieces; what are you going to achieve in the next week or next month? The small wins make the difference.
- Checking in regularly on your progress and acknowledging how far you've come. Recognising progress and success triggers a response in your brain along the lines of, "Ooh, I've achieved something, that's rewarding!" Guess what? Dopamine hit!

- Being prepared to tweak and adjust as you go, rather than sticking rigidly to a goal your brain isn't convinced you will achieve.
- Being kind to your brain and working with it. For example, rather than setting a goal to lose 20 kilograms, have a goal to lose one kilogram in one month's time and have a plan for how you'll achieve it.

**Find out more about Dr Jenny Brockis and her programs at www.drjennybrockis.com**

# Anything is possible

**Mike**

Insane as it sounded, I'd made the decision to get on the Australian team and I was serious about giving it a good go.

It wasn't just a matter of saying "I'm going to be on the team." I needed to break it down into the specific actions that would get me there.

I researched the selection criteria and discovered that only two people from each age group would be chosen to represent Australia at the world championships. This was later extended to three, but at the time I based my approach on being one of two people selected. As I've previously mentioned, the fifties category is very hotly contested.

I asked myself what, specifically, I had to do to make the team. It required an 18-month plan. I worked out that between now and team selection, there would be 12 races where the results would make a difference. Basically, I had to compete in as many races as possible and be on the podium at the end of each of them.

If that wasn't a tall enough order, the races would be held at locations all over Australia.

I've found with any decision to accomplish anything, it's a good idea to think about something you've already achieved, no matter how small it is. That gives you a track record to call on. If you excelled at that one thing, you know you can reach your next goal. Even though this sport was very different to motorbikes, I was able to draw on some of my riding achievements to keep my determination fuelled.

There was a clear picture in my mind of the steps I needed to conquer to get onto that team. This time I wasn't approaching them like that damaged guy pretending to climb the steps at Kings Canyon. This was for real.

I wanted to be coached by the best and was able to work with Tim Jacobs, a former Olympian and the current Australian Olympic kayak coach, who drilled me on technique.

Other members of the paddling community were also incredibly supportive. The reigning world champion in my age group, Mike Mills-Thom, was extremely generous with his time and advice even though I was effectively competing against him for a spot on the Australian team. The women's open world champion, Hayley Nixon from South Africa, who I'd met at various races, couldn't have been more generous and even came to Wollongong to run a training clinic.

I continued to learn from paddling legends like Dean Gardiner, Oscar Chalupsky and Dawid Mocke—even by studying their YouTube videos I always learned something new about technique or race strategy.

Some of the most experienced and awarded members of the Wollongong paddling group also gave me their time and expertise, even though me getting on the national team must have seemed a stretch to them. Champion paddler Cade Barnes took me through coaching sessions on his paddling machine as well as on the water. Other local legends of the sport, Rob Barry and Ian Kennerley, ran a session for me on how to wash-ride, which is similar to drafting on a push bike.

On top of the expert coaching, I went back to the Institute of Sport, under much happier circumstances than my previous visit. I saw an exercise physiologist, who gave me exercises to help my hips and strengthen my back.

I got up early every morning to train; sometimes on the water and on other days—when the ocean conditions weren't right—on a paddling machine I had set up in our downstairs rumpus room. I was also doing regular gym sessions. Any social arrangements were put on hold because I was in bed and asleep by nine o'clock each night, including weekends.

My diet had to change; I made sure I was eating very cleanly with minimal processed food and reduced alcohol.

Every day meant a step closer to my end game; getting onto that team. It wasn't something I just said and left out in the ether. I took daily action.

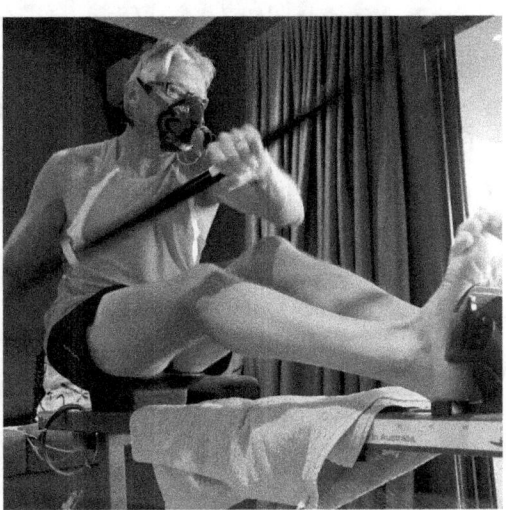

*Off-water training to focus on technique*

In the months leading up to the team selection, I raced in Queensland, Western Australia and all over New South Wales. I entered as many races as I could and went as hard as I was able. As Neryl likes to say, if there'd been a prize for just turning up, I would have got it.

It's probably no surprise that the more I raced, the better I got. Every time I competed, I gained more experience in specific aspects such as how to start strongly.

I had a few shocking race starts along the way, including one occasion when another paddler came off his ski on a wave in front of me and his boat flipped in the air and crashed on me, knocking me into the water. I lost my paddle and was washed back to the beach. I then had to swim several hundred metres to retrieve the boat and start the race all over again.

I also learned more about strategy during a race and how to manage my energy to the finish. I was hanging out with the best paddlers in Australia and got to know many of them and analyse their techniques.

I built a real momentum, and my overall results were good enough to put me second on the ladder for my age group, one place behind multiple world champion Dean Gardiner.

That outcome—way beyond my expectations—gave me a huge amount of confidence.

Knowing the championships would be in Hong Kong in 2017, at the end of 2016 I travelled there on a reconnaissance mission. I competed in a race on the actual championship course, just for practice. There were 150 people in the event, and I won my age group. Now I felt like I was getting somewhere!

I returned to Australia, and the nervous wait began as the selectors made their decision.

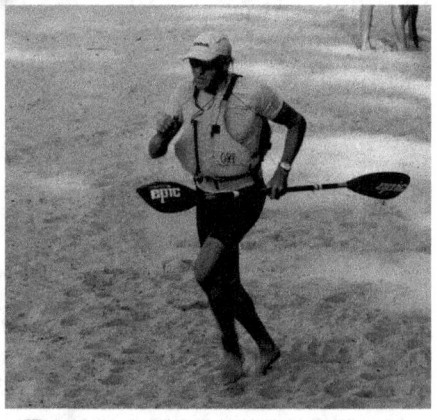

Michael McKeogh I did the same race last year but hobbled up the beach using the paddle as a crutch.
It is so nice having legs that work again 😊

*Even my beach finishes were improving.*

Then, it happened. The Australian team list came out and my name was on it. The diet went out the window that night—a bottle of very good champagne was uncorked.

## 10 | Anything is possible

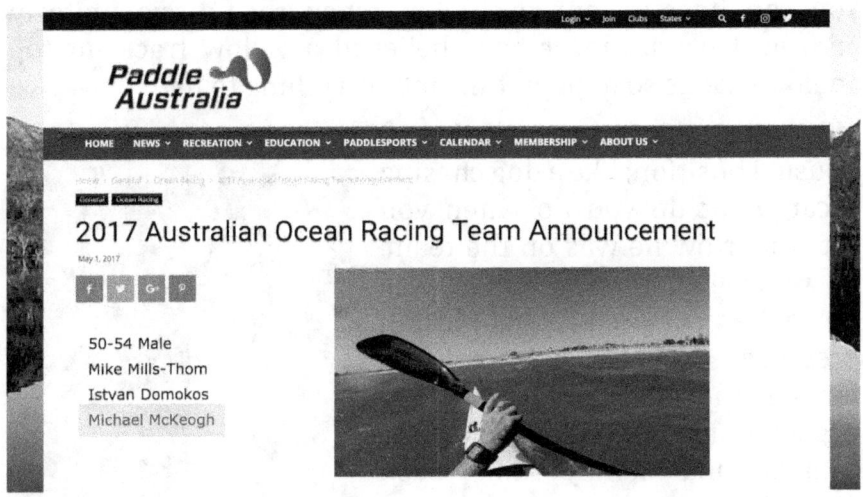

What had been a crazy idea had led to this incredible result. Achieving a goal that once seemed unattainable was truly life changing.

## Neryl

Watching Mike's journey—from the day he declared his intention to get onto that team until the joyous moment when his name was published on the list—was like a master class in how to focus on getting a result.

Yes, he was clear on the target, he broke it down into manageable steps and took action every day. But underpinning that was an unshakeable belief that he *would* get there—even when it seemed impossible.

It's also fascinating to notice that what started as a *giggly goal* became less outrageous over time. That's a key point for all of us; we don't have to settle for the ordinary. Aim for the things that stretch you, that are beyond what you think you can achieve. Then, take daily steps that build your momentum and confidence. You'll find that as you get closer to the result you're seeking, it becomes more realistic.

In the lead-up to the team announcement, we weren't laughing about Mike's goal any more. It was achievable.

You can imagine our excitment when the Aussie uniform arrived. I would never have believed a yellow tracksuit top could make us so happy! It meant everything to us.

Mike now found himself in an unusual position; like a dog chasing a car, what do you do when you catch it? Now he was on the team, he really had to perform. It was no longer a case of him putting pressure on himself without further consequence. He felt the expectations of the team selectors, friends and family and even Australia as a whole, because no-one takes wearing the green and gold lightly.

Just like the saying, there was a whole lot of "bite off more than you can chew, then chew like crazy" going on.

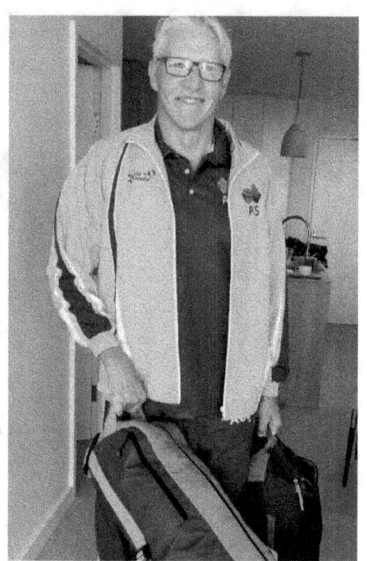

*Looking the part*

For the first time, a sliver of self-doubt found its way in—but that wasn't about to stop Mike.

## Mike

I'd sacrificed a lot to get on the team. I hadn't given my business as much attention as it needed. I didn't spend as much time with my family as I should have. Once the team was announced, I backed off a bit and gave some focus to the things I'd been neglecting. I was still at a very good level of fitness, but the training took a slight back step.

When it got to three months out from the world championships, I needed to put in a major effort. It was a good thing that there were a number of races in Australia leading up to the world event.

I competed in one race, about ten weeks before the championships, and didn't do as well as I expected. That dented my confidence. There was a series of six more races, and I was determined to improve with each event.

I could feel myself getting faster and faster, with incremental improvement in each race. At one event in Newcastle, I chased down and caught a paddler I'd never beaten. Although he held on and crossed the line just ahead of me, he came up and commented on my doggedness in pursuing him throughout the race.

In the final event before I left for Hong Kong, I finished in front of people I hadn't beaten for more than a year. I knew I had prepared myself well; I'd done everything possible to have my best result. I continued to train but also made sure I was well rested.

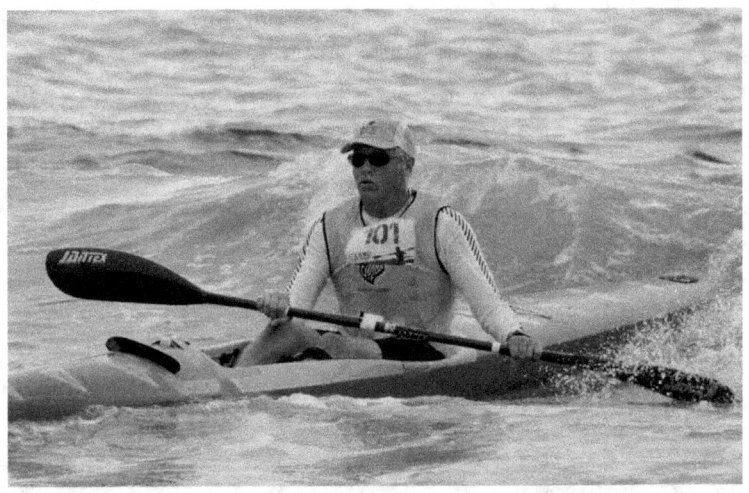

*Countdown to the Championships*

Finally, we arrived in Hong Kong for the world championships. There were more than 300 people from 33 countries to compete against and it was the wildest ocean you've ever seen.

It was what we call a downwind, where the wind is at our back pushing us along. In this case, though, it just whipped up the ocean to a frenzy so there were mountainous seas rather than winds pushing us in the right direction.

But here I was, rubbing shoulders with the best paddlers in the world, each of them champions in their own countries. I'd met many of them at other international events, but this was different. We'd all had to fight for our places in our teams. There was a real sense of this race being "the best of the best".

After everything that had happened to get me there, it was one of those "pinch yourself" moments.

Race day came and we lined up for the start—everyone poised along the beach with waves breaking in front of us. We stood in knee-deep water, waiting for the starting gun. I felt so inadequate, knowing the people on either side of me were champions from America, South Africa and other powerhouse countries of the sport.

The gun fired and it was a frenzy of paddles splashing in the water, trying to get off the line and through the breaking surf. There was carnage on the beach as waves smashed people back on the sand and they lost their boats and paddles. Imagine getting that far, and not getting off the start!

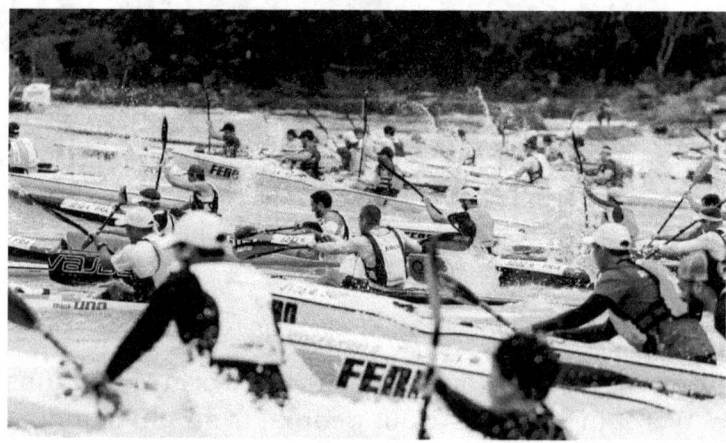

*Start of the World Championships race*

I managed to get going strongly, and the pack headed seven kilometres straight out to sea, with a 30 knot wind hitting us on the side the whole way. The waves broke over our boats and crashed against our sides as we paddled our skinny, six-and-a-half metre long skis into open ocean.

## 10 | Anything is possible

We had to turn around a distant island, so the wind was at our backs for the next 14 kilometres. It was so strong it whipped the ocean into massive peaks, with troughs at least six metres deep.

It was like riding a roller coaster with no way to get off.

Then we turned for home on a four-kilometre stretch of what I hoped was calmer ocean. But the rough conditions meant that even this normally less turbulent section involved rough water and crosswinds.

I got to the finish line, completely unaware of where I'd come in relation to the other paddlers in my age group. Once we turned at the island, the field spread out and it was a lonely paddle home.

I more or less crossed the finish line on my own. There were paddlers immediately in front and behind, but I didn't know what age categories they belonged to.

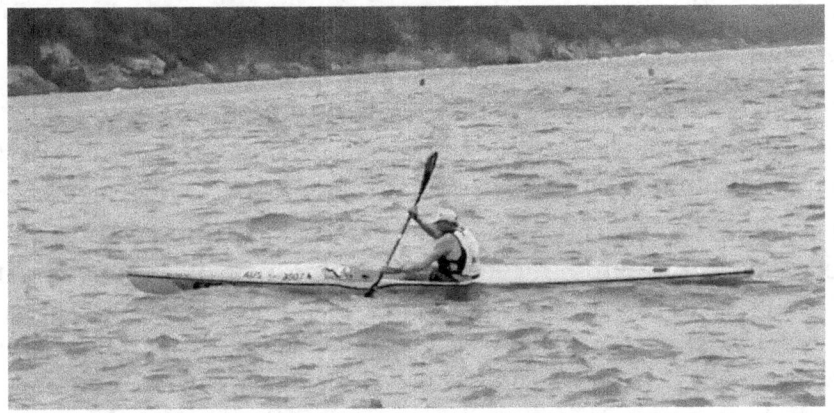

*Finally in the harbour and heading for the finish line*

It was a nail-biting experience for Neryl as a spectator. While she joined the crowd in giving me a huge cheer at the finish, it was impossible to gauge my result. Every competitor looked like a drowned rat wearing fluoro gear and a life jacket.

Still, it felt amazing to have finished a world championship race. I believed I'd done everything I set out to achieve.

There was a long gap between the end of the race and the announcement of the results. Because it was cold and wet, we all took shelter in an indoor basketball court, which was doubling as the registration area and media centre for the championships.

I could see one of the organisers working on the results on his laptop. I was near enough to him to sticky-beak, and for just a second I thought I saw my name come up next to third place.

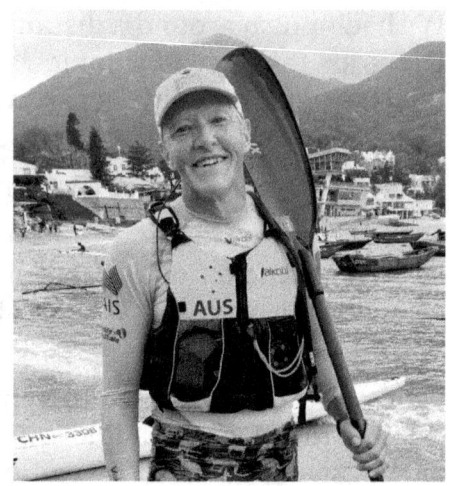

*Finished, exhausted and exultant*

You have to remember, I had no expectation of a podium finish. It was still surreal that I was even there. But over this person's shoulder, it looked like I'd won a bronze medal.

I could see Neryl across the room and I held up three fingers and pointed back to myself. We both shrugged; it seemed too far beyond reality.

I was having an internal battle between absolute, unbridled elation and staying reserved until the awards ceremony, in case I'd read it wrong. I still smarted from an experience at the World Masters Games the year before, when I finished third in a race—and my name was posted as the bronze medallist—only to have another paddler's name called out at the medal ceremony. On that occasion, my backside was already lifted off my seat as I rose to get to the podium, and Neryl was fighting her way to the front with camera poised, only to hear someone else's name. I didn't want a repeat of that experience, so I willed myself not to get my hopes up.

The weather cleared and we went outside for the medal presentations, conducted with full pomp and ceremony and

## 10 | Anything is possible

all the professionalism of an Olympic event. Flags, military, marching music, anthems and the full stage set-up.

We waited while medals were presented in various age groups. The Aussie team had done extremely well across the board. Finally, it was my category's turn.

I was called to the line-up at the side of the stage. I've often joked that it felt like I'd either done something wrong or something very right.

The name of the bronze medallist was called—and it was me.

Next thing, there I was on the podium, receiving a medal at a world championship event.

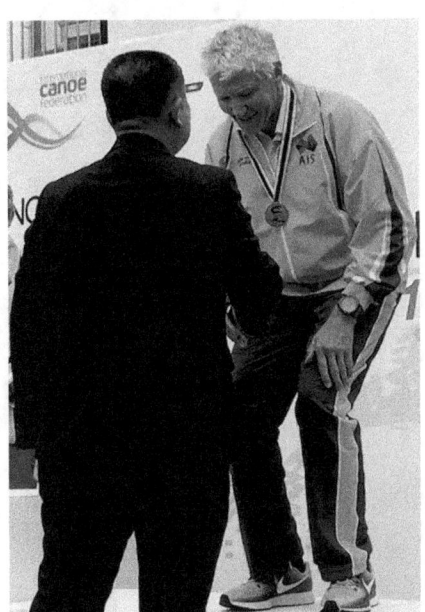 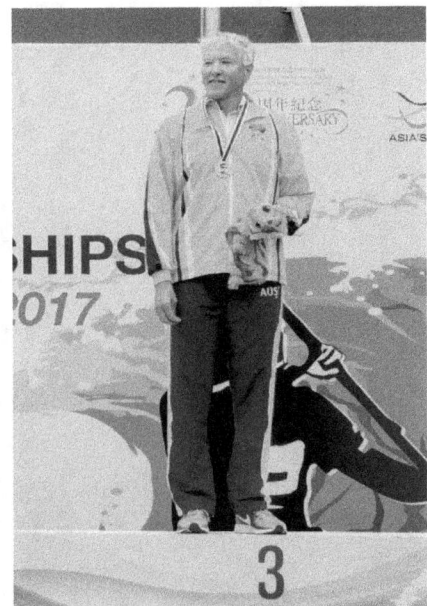

I have to say, being on that stage and bending my head to have the medal hung around my neck was the most incredible feeling. And it wasn't just me receiving this accolade. It was for Neryl, my kids, family, friends and the paddling group in Wollongong who'd supported me through all of it.

I was this guy in a wheelchair just a few years earlier, going from not being able to walk to achieving at a world championship level. It was the most mind-blowing thing in the world.

And after achieving that, anything is possible. Absolutely anything is possible.

# The keys to bouncing back—insights from Sarah Boyd

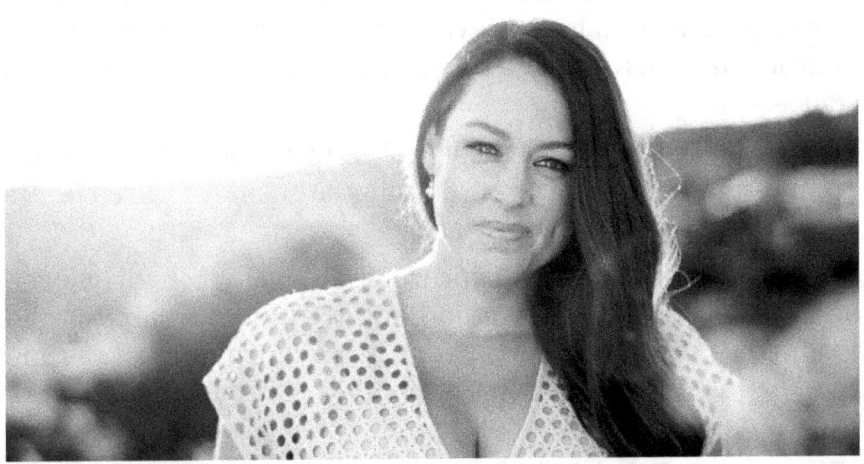

It's normal to feel negative after a negative situation, whether it's a life-changing accident or illness, a financial stress, relationship breakdown or any number of other experiences. While most people go through a slump, certain individuals have the capacity to bounce back to their normal functioning. Studies show some people can actually move on and grow from the experience and they bounce back even higher. This is sometimes called post traumatic coping or growth.

**Sarah Boyd** is an authority on resilience, courage and creativity. She holds a Master of Educational Psychology and a Diploma of

Neuroscience of Leadership. She's also the Founder of *Resilient Little Hearts* Children's Publishing House

As part of the leadership training business Sarah operated with her husband, Colin, she had an understanding—at a logical level—of resilience and how people handle difficult times. One of the core programs Sarah and Colin delivered early in their business was resilience training for organisations, particularly in times of change.

But it was Sarah's personal journey that gave a new perspective on her own level of resilience and the actions she could take in the moment to bounce back, rather than being paralysed by fear or overwhelm.

In her late twenties, with no symptoms or other warnings, Sarah's doctor found a large lump on her neck. After a series of tests she was diagnosed with an aggressive form of thyroid cancer that was already starting to spread into her lymph nodes.

Sarah's life changed radically; going from working full-time, completing her studies and building a business to relentless rounds of radiation and surgery.

Because of the type of cancer Sarah had been diagnosed with, she didn't need chemotherapy. However, her thyroid was removed, and she was set on a lifelong course of thyroid medication that affected her memory, metabolism and general functioning.

"There are whole weeks of treatment that I can't remember because my whole body slowed down," she recalls.

Sarah was in and out of hospital and managing a whirlwind of blood tests, doctors' opinions and check-ups. The treatment lasted 18 months and left her with extreme fatigue. Just as challenging was the psychological impact of going from a driving, ambitious personality to not having the energy to even walk to the letterbox and being bedridden much of the day.

Eventually, Sarah emerged on the other side of her treatment, but another challenge was just around the corner.

"I felt I was really lucky to get to the end of cancer," she says. "I had managed and processed it well, and then we fell pregnant with our first child, Jonah."

"Then I got diagnosed with coeliac disease, an auto-immune condition. Even though it's not life-threatening, because it had been such a short time since my cancer it felt, mentally and emotionally, like I was going through the cancer all over again. It was like, 'It's not fair that I've now got this other chronic condition that I have to manage'."

Over time, Sarah got on top of her coeliac condition, and she and Colin had their second child, Georgia. Towards the end of her pregnancy, she experienced severe pain in her hips.

"I could barely walk, I almost couldn't breathe through the pain. I just thought it was the pregnancy, but after Georgia was born it didn't go away," she remembers.

"They found I had a developmental hip condition that I wasn't aware of. I was born with it but because it wasn't discovered, it was never corrected—so over time my hips had chronically grown out of their sockets. This leads to early onset arthritis in your thirties and real dysfunction around how your muscles grow."

When Georgia was six months old, Sarah had a complete hip replacement on her right side. In time, she'll need similar surgery on her left side.

"In terms of bouncing back, that's where I found it the hardest," she says. "It's one thing to go through one condition for a period of time, but I had now gone through seven years, in and out of chronic conditions that were completely unrelated."

Multiple doctors made the comment to Sarah that they had never seen anyone with so many different health conditions. Mentally, she began to develop what was almost a threat response, continually asking herself what was coming next. A small headache could trigger panic as she questioned what that meant and whether it was a symptom of something serious.

"After that hip diagnosis, I really had to fight for my own power and mental health," she says.

## The steps to Sarah's recovery
*Experiencing all the emotions*

Because of her psychology background, Sarah knew that if she ran away from the experience emotionally, it was going to haunt her by affecting her in other ways. Put simply, she gave herself permission to be however she was in the moment.

"I knew I had to engage with what was happening," she says. "Interestingly, studies show that people who engage with the stressor earlier show more signs of anxiety and depression instantly but are much more likely to see positive growth after the stressor."

*Writing it down*

As an avid journaller, Sarah wrote down everything about her experience and allowed herself to feel all the feelings that were coming and going.

"Journalling has always been something I've used to process events I was going through. Writing is very therapeutic; even if you just write down what you're feeling to get it out and then throw it away. It doesn't have to be a formal journal," she says.

*Defining a bigger purpose*

"I knew I had a purpose that was greater than what I was going through and that this wasn't something I wanted to be defined by at all," says Sarah.

*Seeking and accepting help*

Outside immediate friends, family and medical professionals, Sarah didn't share her story with anyone for three years. She was determined not to be known "as the fragile girl with cancer".

But in terms of seeking support from her inner circle, Sarah didn't hesitate. "I didn't have any shame around it," she says.

## 11 | The keys to bouncing back—insights from Sarah Boyd

"When we went through times when I wasn't feeling like myself, we would go and see a psychologist or friends from church or pastors, and I would be honest with them about how I was feeling."

## How you can build more resilience

While some people seem to have more in-built resilience than others, Sarah believes our early environment and how we each coped with our world as children plays a significant role in our ability to bounce back as adults. As she points out, some people respond to challenging situations from their childhood by developing a deep sense of purpose and needing to move forward, while others crumble under the memories.

A critical factor is how we manage our thinking. Sarah says people who grow through challenges, rather than being defeated by them, share three key factors:

## 1. Resilient people manage meanings effectively

Psychological studies tell us that the impact of an experience has more to do with the *meaning you give it* than the experience itself.

Those who bounce back strongly and grow through negative experiences are generally very good at managing the meaning they put on a situation.

"Two people can go through the same situation, for example a cancer diagnosis; I can make a meaning that cancer is just a hurdle I have to jump over so I can go on and live my best life, and someone else can take the situation to mean that this is the end for them, they must have been cursed to have this happen to them," Sarah says. "The meaning we make largely determines how we handle it."

## 2. Resilient people have "grounded hope"

Sometimes people can put on such a brave face and express so much optimism in terrible circumstances it's apparent their approach is not grounded in reality.

*Grounded hope* is different to optimism. It's an honest understanding of the reality of what you are going through, combined with the ability to continually ask yourself; "Given that I am where I am, how can I still live the best life possible?" Far from being a denial of the situation, it's looking the facts in the face with unwavering hope.

"I still have major limitations in my life, a hundred health appointments that continue even today, but rather than compare myself to someone who doesn't have those things or wonder what life would look like if I didn't have to deal with any of this, I focus on what I've got at the moment, how can I still go on and live the best life for me," says Sarah.

### 3. Resilient people have purpose

People who see growth as a result of challenge feel a purpose in their immediate pain and their life overall. "I know so many things we've done in our business and even me launching a range of children's books have come from that season for me," Sarah explains.

Sarah believes it's important for each of us to build a "resilience bank". When a point of trauma arises in your life, you're then able to draw on what you have invested years before. It's that groundswell of strength that allows you to use the experience to *show* who you are, as opposed to having something negative *define* who you are.

"For someone who's not going through an intense event right now, but they want to build resilience for future events, a lot of it is how we manage our minds and emotions around the daily events we experience," says Sarah.

"Think about building resilience as like strengthening a muscle. You don't want to be going from nothing to heavy weights; you have to build yourself up."

Resilience-building practices include paying attention to the meaning you give to life's everyday challenges, cultivating a community of support around you and considering your higher

## 11 | The keys to bouncing back—insights from Sarah Boyd

purpose; asking yourself what you really want to do with your life.

"Practising those mindset shifts—managing your meaning and emotionally dealing with what is happening in your life, big or small—will set you up for a habit of approaching challenges positively," Sarah says.

"When I was diagnosed with cancer, I didn't suddenly start using resilience tools. I had been implementing them years before."

## Taking responsibility and trusting your gut

Like many people facing health issues, Sarah had to process medical advice from various sources, including opinions that painted a gloomy outlook. She took the approach that you get to decide what the rest of your life is going to be.

"I think it's just deciding that you determine your life," she says.

"With health stuff, you have to take responsibility. Listen to the experts and doctors, and let them help you in the way they can, but at the end of the day it's your body, your health, your life and you have to take responsibility for what you want to see."

"Some people call it belief, some call it faith, others call it the Law of Attraction—it's all about you deciding you're not going to settle for the status quo. You're going to believe something that you don't have physical evidence for at the moment—or you don't have a sign that it's necessarily going to happen for you—but, almost like a bulldog, you are certain, you are set and determined that you're going to see better results than what someone else has told you."

In Sarah's case, an indirect benefit of having so many conditions at once was that she learned not to put too much weight on one individual piece of advice.

"I got to the point where I'd take everyone's opinion with a grain of salt. For example, I had to be on thyroid replacement medication after they removed my thyroid. I would have my

GP call me frantically after a blood test to say my levels were out and that we'd have to make major adjustments, then three hours later I'd have my specialist call and say, 'Oh no, we're in the perfect range for what we need to do.'"

"I was constantly aware that people were just giving their opinions. Yes, they have expertise but they're giving their opinions from their side of the coin. Because I wasn't just dealing with one doctor, I realised I needed to believe what they said, but I was also doing a lot of research myself, and I always trusted my gut—which is so important when you're navigating a thing like that."

Sarah's gut instincts proved correct, time after time. After about 12 months of cancer treatment, it looked like she was going into remission and the end was in sight for her treatment. At the same time, she felt deep down that the treatment wasn't over and there was something wrong. When she went for tests, residual cancer tissue was discovered, and she had to go in for another six months of treatment.

## Finding resilience in the moment

While we can each build resilience over time, what can you do if your life is suddenly disrupted and you can see no immediate way of bouncing back? Here are some quick hacks from Sarah:

**Call a friend.** "I think we rely on ourselves way too much to be positive all the time. I'm very self-reliant and rarely ask for help, but there were times I just needed it. While I was doing everything I knew to manage my head, I actually just needed someone to be encouraging."

**Feel your feelings.** "When you're having a bad day, don't resist it. What often happens is we feel sad or angry or depressed or anxious, and then we put another layer on top that says, 'I shouldn't be feeling this way, what's wrong with me?'"

"I find when you give yourself permission to 'be sad today' or 'feel anxious today', it sometimes releases the whole emotion out of you. Rather than trying to force it, just allow the feelings to come and go."

**Get it out.** "Grab a piece of paper and write out all your feelings. It's very cathartic; if you don't get it out through conversation or writing, it circles in your head and your brain latches onto it—so the best thing you can do is get it out somehow. If you don't have anyone to talk to, just write."

**Find something to be grateful for.** "There's a huge amount of research about gratitude, but it can be extremely difficult to remain grateful while going through a challenge. When I was going through cancer I didn't know anyone else with cancer, and I definitely didn't know anyone my age going through treatment, so it felt very hard at times to do gratitude practice."

"For me, I just made it very small: *I'm grateful I had a good surgeon, I'm grateful they found it when they did.* Those small things begin to snowball."

Be nice to yourself. Do things that make you feel good. "I remember during the treatment all I wanted—because I was inside all day—was to sit in the sun. That was something I focused on doing, to get up from the bed."

"With cancer I had huge fatigue, but I never had physical pain. With my hip, I couldn't sleep at night. Even on heavy drugs I wasn't sleeping. I was a horrible person at home. I was grumpy all the time, snappy at the kids and Colin, and then I felt bad about being like that because I felt like I wasn't being a great wife, mum or friend. I felt like a burden because I was always going through something.

"But, looking back, I wish I was kinder to myself. I really was going through a hectic situation."

**Sarah Boyd is passionate about lifting the limits off an individual's potential so they can pursue their dreams and live a meaningful life. Find out more about Sarah's work at www.sarahboyd.co**

# Disrupting your own life

Each of us will go through challenges of varying degrees; it's part of being human. As you have seen in this story, it's possible to use the momentum of that difficulty to propel you to the next level in your life.

Even better, you don't need to wait until a major problem or negative experience forces you to make changes. You can take the initiative by disrupting your *own* life.

What is it that gets you out of bed every day? Do you have a *giggly goal*? If not, is it time to start believing again that you're capable of anything?

Perhaps you've been trying to make a change for years, like quitting smoking or getting fitter, but you never seem to get there.

Rather than waiting for a major health episode to make the decision for you, you can change your daily choices and actions, and put yourself on the path to a different result. These choices don't have to be huge; it's all about taking one step at a time.

Now that you've read this book, including insights from experts on the subject of *bouncing back*, we'd like to present some thoughts and specific tools that have helped us on our journey since the accident in 2010.

Think of this final chapter as being like a "tasting plate" you might be served in a restaurant; a sampling of the chef's best offerings. Notice which ones resonate for you and consider applying them in your own life.

## Mike

My experience since 2010 has reinforced what I've believed for a long time: If you fix your mind on a clear outcome and make a committed choice to take daily action towards it, you will accomplish more than you could have dreamed.

There were other paddlers in my age group who could have been on that Australian team—stronger and faster competitors than me—but I believe I was the only one who set it as a target and did everything needed to achieve it. That made the difference.

Achieving results isn't necessarily about coming first. I won bronze, not gold, but to me the colour of the medal is irrelevant. It's what it represents that counts. It's proof that I achieved the result I was seeking, and so much more.

We can all create our best life possible, regardless of our circumstances. For you, that might involve achieving something out of the ordinary, or it might be making a small change to your life or commiting to living the best version of it that you can.

Think about your life over the last five years. Does that thought fill you with happiness and satisfaction or negative emotions like disappointment, anxiety or sadness? By looking at your recent history, you'll get a good indication of what your life will probably be like into the future.

That's because by the time we reach adulthood, we're generally set in our ways; making the same kinds of choices and taking similar action every day, mostly on autopilot. Not surprisingly, we get similar results over and over.

If you repeat the same choices thoughout your life, little will change—whether it's your career, business, relationships, finances, health, fitness or any other aspects. On the other hand, if you decide on something different and take the action that heads you in that direction, you're writing yourself a different future.

One of the things I've learned through this experience is that you don't have to just accept what happens to you. You can decide to make something triumphant from the situation, which can be even better than what you had before.

Whatever the life you want to create for yourself, be clear about your decision. Choose to take daily action towards it. And gravitate to those people who will give you all the support you need to get there.

> "Nothing changes if nothing changes" - Unknown

## Own your goals

Before I set up my fibre optics business I had the idea that I wanted to be a teacher at TAFE, the technical and further education system in New South Wales which has equivalents in other Australian states and around the world. I'd done my electrical trade and had worked for many years managing telecommunications projects for large industrial contracting companies. Moving into the education system, where I could help train future fibre optic technicians, seemed a logical step. The pay was reasonable and the conditions were good.

I did the appropriate level of teacher training and became a part-time teacher, gradually taking on more and more hours. When the opportunity arose for a full-time post I sat the exam, went through rounds of interviews and got the job.

I should have been over the moon, but I wasn't. It was only after I was offered the role that I realised this wasn't my dream. It was what my parents had wanted for me. I had made it my mission to get a full-time teaching job and taken all the steps to achieve it, but I didn't *own* the goal. Deep down, it wasn't what I really wanted to do.

In the end, I turned down the job and learned a powerful lesson. We can achieve what we set our mind on but it must be *our* choice, not someone else's.

Whatever outcome you might be seeking, whether it's moving on from a dramatic life disruption or creating a small change in your current circumstances, own it and connect to it with your mind, heart and soul.

## Draw on past achievements

I mentioned earlier in the story that whenever you're trying to achieve anything, whether it's a big goal or a small action, you can call on your past experience at achieving results. It's a point worth emphasising.

Have you previously decided to do something and been able to achieve it? If so, you have a positive track record you can draw on.

For example, many people end up in financial difficulties as a result of going through a divorce. This happened to me when my first marriage ended.

Back in my mid twenties, I was doing well for myself. I owned property, a nice car and regularly travelled overseas. By the time I reached 40, I felt like I'd lost the lot. I was faced with the prospect of starting again from nothing.

That was an extremely difficult time. However, I'd done it once before. Now that I had 15 years of extra experience on the clock, I knew I could do it again and better—and I did. I drew on my previous achievements and experience, and built my finances up beyond what they were before.

You can take this principle and apply it to any area of your life.

## Set micro goals that keep you moving

As Allan Parker described in Chapter 7, the choices you make *right now*, not later today or next week, are the ones that count the most. For me, this means being able to break down large tasks or challenges into tiny, achievable pieces. If you can do that, you're far less likely to get thrown off course at the first obstacle.

I remember competing in a paddling marathon and being completely exhausted after the first half of the race. I really didn't want to go on. The voice in my head was screaming "STOP! There's nothing left in the tank!"

In that moment, I could either listen to that voice or take control and lead the way.

To get to the end of the event, I created a series of micro goals of between 30 seconds and a minute. In my exhausted state, that timeframe was all I could wrap my mind around. I knew I could hang on for another minute, but if I'd thought to myself, "There's another hour and a half of this to get through," I would have given up.

Great things begin with small steps. I got through the next 30 seconds... and felt a sense of achievement. I didn't have time to celebrate because I was still in the middle of a race, but I'd reached my immediate goal. I believe the ability to notice your small achievements while continually moving forward is the secret to success.

I got through the next 30 seconds and the one after that, then another. Before I knew it, I was crossing the finish line!

I didn't beat my best time, but I finished what I started. In doing so, I gave myself another positive experience to draw on.

I believe this is what stops most people from achieving great things. They set their sights high, then get stuck and stop in their tracks. They don't know how to create new, smaller goals to build their confidence back up so they can move on to bigger and better things.

## Don't "set and forget"

Being clear about what you want to achieve, whether large-scale or small, and visualising what your life will be like when you get there, is a powerful way to set you up for success.

However, a positive mindset is just the start. You must consciously take steps every single day towards your goal.

When I wanted to get onto the Australian team, I didn't simply set the goal and forget about it. I certainly cultivated a positive belief that I would make the team, but I also broke it down into specific actions and completed each task.

That pattern of completion helped me gather momentum which, in turn, gave me the impetus to keep going. My desired result got closer every day until I could almost reach out and touch it.

## When you don't want to do it, do it anyway

Having a clear mental picture of your result helps override the way you might feel in a specific moment. This applied to me many times, especially when I didn't want to get up early for training or travel a long distance to a race.

Focusing on your end game, rather than the reasons for not continuing, makes it easier to overcome your own objections. Your commitment to taking the action is so strong you stop listening to your inner complaint system.

## Focus on others

Related to the previous point, you'll have even more reason for continuing towards your desired result if it's more about *other people* than you.

In previous chapters I described how, during my recovery, I focused on being the best partner and parent I could be. I knew my accident had a profound impact on my family, so I wanted to recover for them. I continually asked myself, "Who do I need to be for the people who need me?" I turned my focus outwards, as Allan Parker describes in Chapter 7. This gave me so much more motivation than if I had been thinking solely of my own wellbeing.

Consideration of others gives us powerful reasons to behave differently. Think of a child suddenly crying out in the middle of the night. A sleeping parent will wake up immediately and go to the child. No matter how tired the parent feels, they'll get out of bed.

What changes would you like to make in your life, whether significant or small? Who else will benefit from these changes? Focus on *them* as the main reason for moving towards your goal.

A good example of this is someone struggling to improve their fitness or general health. Perhaps they've tried for years to lose weight or get motivated enough to do regular exercise. Focusing on other people can be the fuel that powers up that missing motivation. If the person has children or grandchildren, being fitter and healthier will make it easier to play with the kids, creating stronger bonds and special memories. By improving their health they'll be becoming the best partner they can be for their spouse, boyfriend or girlfriend, which will have all manner of pleasurable side effects including in the bedroom. If they don't have a partner and want to find one, their newer, fitter self will have increased confidence in the dating arena. If they're happy being single, new-found fitness will make them a more effective manager, employee, team member, aunt, uncle... you can fill in the blanks.

## Accept it won't be easy

Any change can be challenging because our brains are wired to keep things the way they are. If you're going for a large-scale change or a significant achievement, the challenge is even more intense. It's important to be real about it; there will be internal conflict. Your mind will give you a thousand reasons why you should give up. Most of us are experts at self-sabotage.

Recognise that, and move on. Realise that we all face obstacles to what we want to achieve; they are part of the journey.

In my case, it wasn't always easy to make decisions about my recovery after the accident. At times it was very hard to disregard medical advice, especially when so many doctors were telling me my life would never be the same, "this is your lot". It was difficult to keep going in the face of those comments, even if I didn't accept them.

Some medical professionals began blaming me, implying I was a hypochondriac for continually complaining about the pain I felt and insisting they do something about it. They weren't used to having a patient who refused to accept their prognosis. The kilos and kilos of X-rays in my cupboards are testament to the fact that no-one could work it out, until I finally found the right person who listened to me.

So, accept it won't be easy. Don't let that be the reason you don't succeed.

> "Only those who will risk going too far can possibly find out how far one can go." – T. S. Eliot

## Sell yourself the upside

Most life disruptions involve a degree of fear and discomfort. Regardless of what you're shooting for, for example weight loss, a better relationship or business growth, ask yourself, "What's the upside of this change?" and then sell yourself that idea.

Consider what the change will cost you. Then do a simple version of a cost-benefit analysis: do the benefits outweigh the cost? If the answer is yes, you now have a compelling upside. You've identified why it's worth going through that particular change.

You can use that to override your inbuilt self-protection system and stretch yourself out of your comfort zone.

Before the accident, I knew I had a good life. Being on walking sticks, in constant pain and not being able to run was not the life I wanted to live. My upside to pushing through the pain and persevering with treatment after treatment was getting my norm back, and I was very convincing in selling that to myself.

Going for the Australian team took this concept to a whole different level. Now it was pushing myself to take on rigorous training, change my diet and complete a hectic schedule of gruelling races. The whole idea was a huge stretch.

I sold it to myself by focusing on the sense of accomplishment I knew would be waiting at the other end. To go from being so broken to getting onto an Australian team would be remarkable by anyone's standards, and in my mind that would make it worthwhile. Such an achievement would defy those years of advice from doctors and psychiatrists and be beyond all expectations, including my own.

What's the upside of your change or desired achievement? Keep that in your mind at all times.

> "Pearls don't lie on the seashore. If you want one, you must dive for it." – Chinese proverb

## Neryl

Of course, your desired outcome doesn't have to involve getting onto a national team for a global sporting event. You can choose to disrupt your life in any number of ways that are significant to you. It might be committing to go for a walk every day, being more assertive in meetings at work or keeping in regular contact with family members.

Whatever it is, it's the combination of having the *will* to do it and then taking the *action* that gets the result.

My targets are relatively small, including drinking a certain amount of water each day. In the past, I often forgot to drink enough water and found myself dehydrated. This small commitment has made a big difference to my health.

Another of my desired outcomes is to spend time with friends, ideally in person but at least on the phone, every week. Without that specific commitment I could easily find myself absorbed in work and not take the time to catch up with people important to me.

Simple steps can make a profound difference.

Here are some ideas and resources that have helped me, both through the difficult times after Mike's accident and more recently as we continue to build an outstanding future.

## Aim for a calm mind

Going through a life disruption, especially one that's not of your choosing, can be overwhelming. Hopefully one of your takeaways from our story is the power of the human mind, even in the most challenging circumstances. Whatever happens, we always get to choose our response.

It's not always easy to remember that principle, especially in very emotional or stressful situations. Like many people around the world, I have found huge benefit in meditation. If you haven't tried meditation you might think it's complicated or difficult, but that isn't the case.

My go-to meditation app is *Headspace*, which is accurately marketed as "meditation made simple". Downloading this app and using it for a few minutes each day can have a huge impact on your overall level of calmness and clarity.

Another favourite is *The Honest Guys* on YouTube, which provides guided meditations ranging in length from a few minutes to eight hours. You'll find them at www.youtube.com/user/TheHonestGuys

There are many other meditation options, from groups and retreats to online courses—or you could just sit in a quiet place for a few moments and concentrate on taking deep breaths.

Whatever works best for you, spend time each week on activities that build your resilience reserves, especially if you're supporting someone else in a crisis situation.

## Your own truth counts

There were many times when Mike's recovery and, later, his determination to succeed in his sport could have been derailed by the beliefs of others. With the best intentions, people commented to me about how Mike's long-term injuries would affect the quality of my life and our future together.

What others present as "truth" is really their opinion, belief or interpretation of available information. It's their version of the truth but it isn't necessarily accurate. You know, deep down, what you're capable of, regardless of the circumstances around you. In our situation, we had our own version of the truth and we stuck to it.

I heard some great advice recently about not taking another person's feedback to heart unless they're in the arena with you, experiencing everything you're experiencing. I've since found this helpful in many different contexts.

When you're making any kind of change, others will inevitably give their advice. By all means listen politely, especially if it's well-intended. But remind yourself that you get to decide your next move.

## Don't just do it, *be* it

In our conference presentations, we speak a lot about being *clear on the vision* of what you want to achieve, *making the decision* to go for it and taking the *specific, daily actions* that will get you there.

For that combination to really kick into gear, you must fuel it with unstoppable belief. Rather than just doing the steps and going through the motions, you need to *be* the person who will achieve that specific result.

In Mike's case, he had to become a world-championship-standard athlete, despite the fact that when he started, he was a long way from his goal. He had to imagine himself already being selected onto the national team and choose the thoughts and actions that an athlete of that calibre would demonstrate.

I recently heard a presentation by champion modern pentathlete Chloe Esposito, who won gold in her sport at the Rio Olympics. Her whole journey to Olympic glory was inspiring, from her decision to take up the sport to her various successes and how she bounced back after injury and disappointment.

What particularly resonated with me was her description of the final event in the gruelling Rio modern pentathlon, the combined running and shooting. At the start of that round, Chloe was seventh in the field with a 45-second handicap.

There was a moment when she was suddenly fired up with determination. In that second she *became* a gold medallist; she knew, to the very core of her being, that she would take the lead and win the pentathlon.

Her competitors faltered during the last round of shooting and she was suddenly able to pull away for the final run leg. Even though she'd gone into that final event as the underdog, Chloe not only won gold but set a new Olympic record in the sport.

Brain science expert Jim Fortin speaks about this in his weekly podcast, *Transform Your Life from the Inside Out*. Whatever change you want to introduce into your life, from being more organised to giving up smoking and everything in between, Jim argues that nothing will alter until you change who you are *being*. If you're frequently late and disorganised, you need to *be* a person who is organised and punctual. To successfully quit, the smoker must *be* a person who is a non-smoker, rather than a smoker trying to give up cigarettes.

During Mike's recovery, I became a carer. It's not that I ever had any desire to be one or any idea how to do it well. I just made a decision, at a very deep level, to be his primary carer. That enabled me to put everything else aside, for that time, and focus on looking after Mike and the kids. I committed to being the best carer and stepmother I could possibly be.

A powerful piece of advice I've received is to write down my intentions each morning for who I will *be* that day. This is not a to-do list or a series of general, positive affirmations. It's four or five specific statements about the person I will be over the next 24 hours; for example, "I am a person who is focused and effective," "I am the CEO of a thriving business," or "I am a calm and patient listener today."

Over time, I've noticed subtle differences in my thought processes, decisions and general approach, aligned with my stated intentions.

This is easy to do and fun to experiment with. Who are you being today?

## Re-record your inner conversations

To fully take on the belief that you are now a person who achieves (insert your desired result here), you might need to have a frank discussion with the voice in your head that brings up all the reasons why you won't succeed.

The conversations you have with yourself are the most important interactions of all; they drive your beliefs and emotions. If your thoughts are constantly at odds with what you're trying to achieve, you're in danger of caving in to self-sabotage.

As well as the specific intentions I referred to in the previous section, I've found it very helpful to use affirmations to lay a foundation of positive thought in my mind.

Affirmations are simply positive statements you say about yourself or your situation. They can be specific, but you can also use more general affirmations about areas of your life such as success, health, love, money etc. By repeating these statements, you're aiming to influence both your conscious and subconscious mind.

Most of us have a continual loop of inner dialogue playing in our head, and it's usually negative and self-critical. Affirmations are a way of replacing that trashy self-talk with uplifting, positive words. Over time, if we practise them often enough, those statements become our new habitual self-talk.

Even though I speak on stages for a living, in the past I lacked confidence and allowed poor self-belief to hold me back in various areas of my life. I learned about the power of affirmations after I reached a particularly low point. I began saying a simple affirmation, "I approve of myself," hundreds of times a day. I'd say it out loud when I could, or if I was in public, I'd say it to myself over and over again.

The results were dramatic. Within a few weeks I felt differently about myself. Friends began to notice a positive change and commented on it. To say that short statement changed my life sounds melodramatic, but it's true. I still use it today if I have a moment when my self-belief temporarily deserts me.

To give your affirmations extra punch, try standing in front of a mirror, looking yourself directly in the eyes and saying your statements aloud. I challenge you to do it the first time without laughing or criticising yourself for some perceived flaw. Stick with it, and you might just notice a shift in your thoughts, feelings and behaviour.

There are many excellent books on how to reprogram your inner dialogue using affirmations and other tools. One of my favourites is Dr Joe Dispenza's *Breaking the Habit of Being Yourself* (www.drjoedispenza.com).

> "The successful warrior is the average man, with laser-like focus." - Bruce Lee

## Dismantle unhelpful beliefs in the moment

Even after trying all the tools we've suggested, a life disruption can have us responding in all kinds of negative ways. What I've learned is that often we're not responding to the actual *event* that's happened; we're responding to the *story* we're telling ourselves about the event.

If you're trying to achieve a certain result and something throws you off target, it can be easy to take that situation and give it a negative, personal spin; such as, "I'll never be able to do this", or "I knew this would be too hard." That story, in turn, creates a negative emotion which might lead you to react more strongly than if you had been responding to the original situation alone.

When you feel that negative emotion rising, it can be really useful to ask yourself whether you're reacting to a *fact* or a *story*. Just checking in with yourself can make a big difference. It also gives you the opportunity to make a different choice about what you do next.

Neuropsychologist Dr Shannon Irvine (www.drshannonirvine.com) recommends taking your negative story or belief and putting it on trial in an imaginary courtroom, then dismantling it as if you were the world's best attorney cross-examining a hapless witness. Does your story have any factual supporting evidence? Is there evidence (and there usually is) that shows your belief to be false? Have you ever heard of anyone else achieving what you're trying to do? If so, it's not an impossible challenge.

Another effective way of looking at your beliefs at moments when you're tempted to give up on a goal is to choose to replace your current thought with something more *useful*. Speaker and author Chris Helder (www.chrishelder.com) argues that useful beliefs are more effective than "positive thinking", which can be a stretch when you're in a negative situation.

Rather than trying to force yourself to hold onto a cheery thought when you confront an obstacle, Helder's philosophy is about having belief systems that support you. He recommends asking yourself questions like, "What's the most useful thing to believe about this situation?" and "What is the most useful thing I could do today to get me closer to where I want to be?"

The interesting thing is, your belief doesn't have to be *true* in that moment. It just needs to be more useful than the negative thought you were thinking.

## Have a framework for your goals

Doing the inner work is critical, but you've probably gathered by now that we're also strong believers in the power of taking action. Those two approaches—mind and deed—work hand in hand.

When it comes to the action side of the equation, many people say they're going to achieve goals or change habits, but their enthusiasm wanes after a short time and they stop doing what's necessary. I've found having a written framework makes a huge difference in keeping me on target with my actions.

There are many approaches to this, from online products and apps to hard-copy planners. It's important to use the one that feels right for you.

For me, the key is to keep it simple. At the start of each year I spend a short amount of time thinking about where I want to be at the end of the next 12 months, across all areas of my life. You could choose the headings most relevant for you; I generally focus on:

- Business
- Relationships
- Health/fitness
- Spiritual
- Finances

From there, I write down the specific actions needed over the next year to get to my desired result. Some outcomes will require a number of different actions, while others need only one.

Then I prioritise; realistically, I'm not going to take *all* the actions I've listed so I choose my top eight. I create a table in a Word document (I told you I like simplicity!), with nine columns. The heading for the first column is *Action*. The next seven columns have headings for the seven days of the week. The ninth column is titled *Progress*.

I then populate the first column with my eight actions and away I go! Each afternoon I jot down a few notes to record the specific actions I've taken that day. Some of these are tiny, like sending a particular email or speaking to someone.

At the end of the week I give myself a G, A or R (green, amber or red) in the *Progress* column for each of my eight actions. I can see at a glance how I'm tracking. I save the file under that week's date range and start a new document for the next week.

Every three months I review my actions to see if I need to make any changes. Sometimes I delete an action if it's been sitting in "red" for a number of weeks and I know, deep down, I'm not really committed to it. I might do some tweaking or add something completely new.

This whole process only takes a matter of minutes each day, but the results have been significant. Rather than feeling overwhelmed by the number of tasks I'm confronted with each morning, I know exactly where to put my focus if I want to progress my goals. I find I am so much more productive, and I've had the satisfaction of achieving many of my desired results.

For example, as a professional speaker I had a long-held desire to become a Certified Speaking Professional (CSP), which is an international designation achieved by only a small percentage of people in my profession.

Looking at the criteria as a whole, it seemed daunting and out of my reach. But by breaking it down into specific actions and following this process over several years, I gradually moved closer to my goal. Just as Mike got momentum as he took daily steps towards getting onto the Australian ocean racing team, I could feel my result becoming more and more realistic.

When I was awarded my CSP designation in 2017 it felt like a completely natural progression. I'd set the vision, made the decision to achieve it and taken the small steps that eventually got me there.

Whatever process you use, the magic happens when you get clear, specific and action-focused.

## Be accountable

Sometimes it's not enough to keep yourself accountable, even by writing down your actions each day. That's when you need to call for reinforcements, enlisting the support of other people to keep you on track.

Support could be in the form of a fitness coach, relationship counsellor, business adviser or other professional. Or it could be a less formal arrangement; for example, I'm part of a small group of fellow speakers/entrepreneurs who meet monthly with the specific aim of keeping each other accountable on our business journey. This has been extremely useful in clarifying my goals and getting support and feedback on my progress.

Family and friends can also be great supporters and sounding boards; just remember to treat any negative feedback with respectful caution, especially if they don't fully understand the context of your goals.

> "Our destiny is not written for us, it's written by us."
> –Barack Obama

## And finally...

*Disrupt Your Life* is a story about rising above a challenge and achieving something extraordinary. There are countless other inspirational stories online, in bookstores and libraries to help keep you focused on what you can achieve, regardless of your circumstances.

We hope this chapter, in particular, has given you some ideas and resources to help you bounce back in any situation. You might like to jot down your own ideas on the remaining pages.

Wherever you are right now, you already have everything you need to achieve what you want in your life, from the extraordinary to the everyday. Make the choice and go for it.

**What will you achieve when you make the decision to disrupt your life?**

## A place to record your *giggly goals* and actions

# About the authors

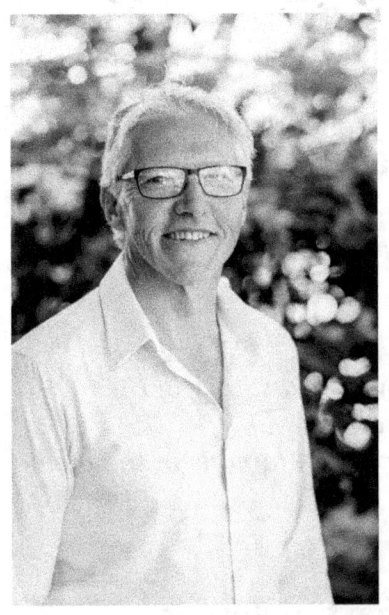

**Michael McKeogh** is an award-winning business owner and entrepreneur. After a diverse career path that included electrician, police officer, tourist coach driver, immigration consultant, garbage collector and telecommunications project manager, Mike started his company, Fibre Optics Design and Construct, on his dining room table.

It has since been a pivotal part of some of Australia's biggest infrastructure projects and achieved national acclaim in the electrical and communications industry.

In 2010, Mike suffered critical leg and spinal injuries in a motorbike accident and was faced with the prospect of never walking properly again. Defying medical opinions, Mike not only recovered but set his sights on competing for Australia in his newly-adopted sport, surf ski paddling.

He exceeded all expectations by winning bronze for Australia at the 2017 World Ocean Racing Championships in Hong Kong.

**Dr Neryl East** is a communication and credibility expert who shows leaders and teams how to stand out, accelerate their success and avoid costly reputation mistakes.

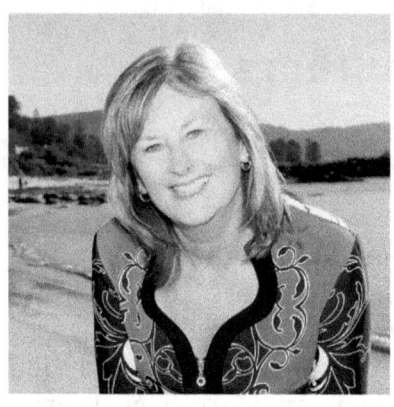

Neryl has been a professional communicator for more than three decades, including a career in television and radio and a stint as an Olympic announcer. She has also spent many years managing high-profile issues in the public and private sectors, and training executives and entrepreneurs on leading in the media spotlight.

Neryl has a PhD in Journalism, is a Certified Speaking Professional and an Amazon best-selling author on media and reputation.

Other titles by Dr Neryl East:

- *Named and Shamed: Rod Oxley's Inside Story of the Wollongong Corruption Scandal*
- *The Headline Edge: How you can get famous in the media through free PR*

Visit www.neryleast.com

## Book us as speakers for your next conference

If you were inspired by our story in *Disrupt Your Life,* help us share this important message with an even bigger audience by engaging us to speak at your next conference or event.

Our powerful keynote presentation makes audiences think differently about their life and career. After hearing our experience, they realise they can, at any time, disrupt their own life.

*About the authors*

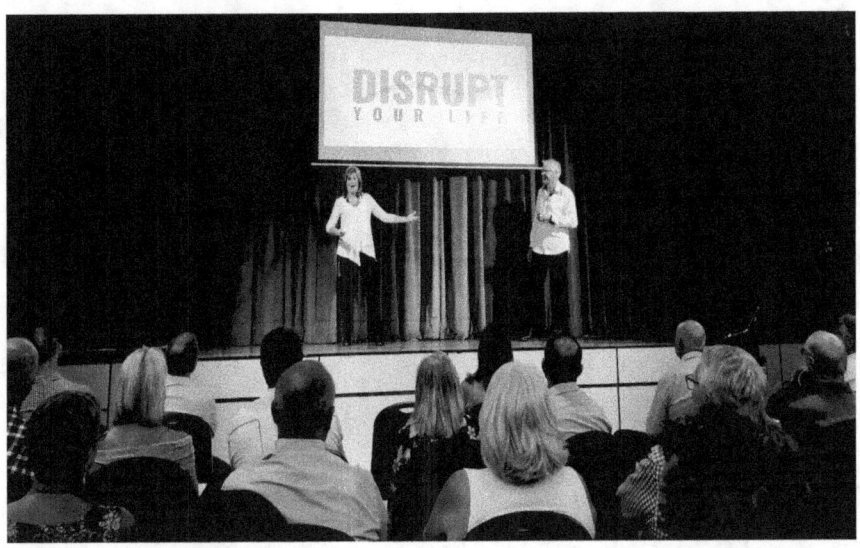

**What audiences say:**

"You need to hear this story - it has so much inspiration. It makes you believe in taking hold of your life." - Amanda Floyd

"This is a story about turning ordinary into extraordinary." - Anne Goodall

"If you are looking for some inspiration and practical advice on how to overcome adversity, this is for you!" - James Hale

Visit www.disruptyourlife.com.au

**Want even more help creating your vision and achieving your goals? Join us for a Total Focus workshop.**

Achieving extraordinary results starts with your daily decisions and actions. Getting total focus, so you become crystal clear on your goals and know exactly what to do to achieve them, can be as simple as following a proven process.

Total Focus is one of a powerful suite of programs delivered in conjunction with YB12 (Your Best 12 Months). See the details at www.yb12coach.com and contact us at info@neryleast.com for information about upcoming programs, including online options.

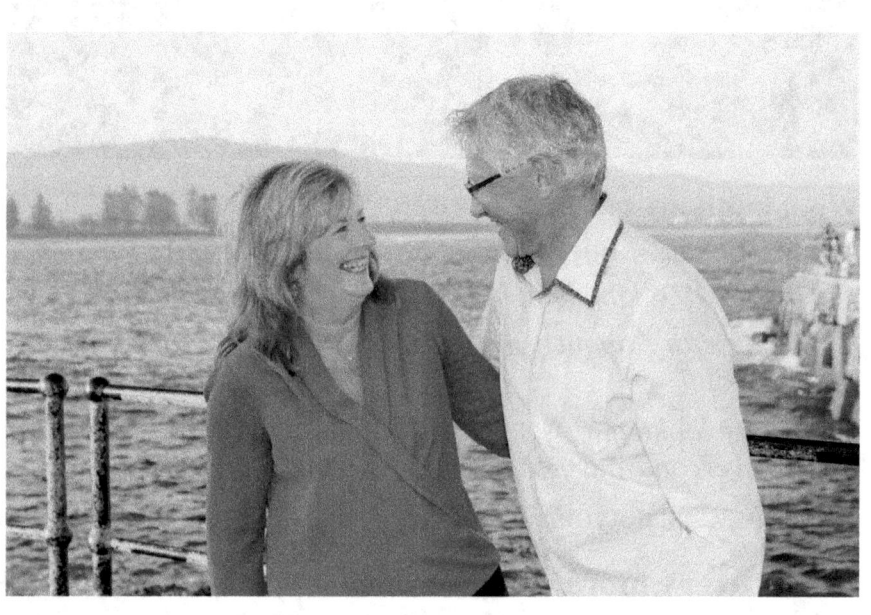

www.ingramcontent.com/pod-product-compliance
Lightning Source LLC
Chambersburg PA
CBHW070607010526
44118CB00012B/1467